Girls in Trouble

By the Same Authors

Sin in the City: Sexuality and Social Control in Urban Scotland, 1660–1780
Leah Leneman and Rosalind Mitchison
1 898218 90 0

Girls in Trouble

Sexuality and Social Control in Rural Scotland 1660–1780

Rosalind Mitchison and Leah Leneman

SCOTTISH CULTURAL PRESS
EDINBURGH

Published in 1998 by
Scottish Cultural Press
Unit 14, Leith Walk Business Centre
130 Leith Walk, Edinburgh EH6 5DT
Tel: 0131 555 5950 • Fax: 0131 555 5018
e-mail: scp@sol.co.uk

Copyright © Rosalind Mitchison and Leah Leneman 1998

This is a revised edition of *Sexuality and Social Control: Scotland 1660–1780*,
first published by Blackwells in 1989

*All rights reserved. No part of the publication may be reproduced,
stored in a retrieval system, or transmitted in any form or by any
means, electronic, digital, mechanical, photocopying, recording or
otherwise, without prior permission of Scottish Cultural Press*

British Library Cataloguing in Publication Data
A catalogue record for this book is available from the British Library

ISBN: 1 898218 89 7

Printed and bound by
Interprint Ltd, Malta

Contents

List of Figures		vi
List of Tables		vi
Acknowledgements		vii
List of Abbreviations		viii
	Introduction	1
1	The Scottish Church	5
2	The Changing Economic and Social Setting	20
3	Regular Marriage	40
4	Irregular Marriage	53
5	Patterns in Illegitimacy and Pre-marital Conceptions	72
6	Where, When and Why	91
7	Response to Authority	106
	Conclusion	122
Appendix: a list of parishes used for quantitative work		127
Index		128

List of Figures

5.1	Scottish illegitimacy ratios, national sample	75
5.2	Illegitimacy ratios: Lothians, Fife and Central Lowlands	76
5.3	Illegitimacy ratios: Western Highlands, Central and Eastern Highlands	76
5.4	Illegitimacy ratios: Aberdeenshire, the North-east and Caithness	77
5.5	Illegitimacy ratios: Ayrshire and the South-west	77

List of Tables

4.1	Irregular marriages registered after the event	56
4.2	Irregular marriages as percentage of total marriages	58
5.1	Sample calculation: Central Lowlands 1761–1770	74
5.2	Illegitimacy ratios: 1760s and 1858–1860	75
5.3	Illegitimacy ratios: Westerkirk and the South-west	78
5.4	Time of discovery of antenuptial conception (%)	85

Acknowledgements

The research on which this book is based has been supported by the Economic and Social Research Council (at that time the Social Science Research Council), the British Academy and the Leverhulme Trust. We are grateful to these organisations for making the study possible, and to the Department of Economic and Social History of Edinburgh University which has provided us with space, secretarial aid and the miscellaneous support and encouragement which counts for a great deal in the carrying on of a research project.

Most of the material used was located in the Scottish Record Office, and we have benefited from the courtesy and expertise of the staff. We are also grateful for the help of the staffs of the National Library of Scotland and of the regional archives in Forres, Dundee, Stirling and Glasgow.

Individuals to whom we owe ideas, suggestions, information and general help include Michael Anderson, R.H. Campbell, Tristram Clarke, Michael Lynch, Rosalind Marshall, Rory Paddock, Geoffrey Parker, Alasdair Roberts, David Sellar, T.C. Smout, I.A. Whyte and E.A. Wrigley.

The text for this revised edition was much improved by the editorial hand of Graham Sutton.

Abbreviations

APS   *Acts of the Parliaments of Scotland,* 12 vols. (London, 1814–75).
KSR   Kirk Session Register.
NLS   National Library of Scotland.
NSA   *New Statistical Account of Scotland,* 15 vols. (Edinburgh, 1845).
OPR   Old Parish Register.
OSA   *The Statistical Account of Scotland,* Sir John Sinclair (ed.), 21 vols. (Edinburgh, 1791–97): revised in a regional arrangement with introductions in 20 vols., Donald J. Withrington and Ian R. Grant (eds.), (Wakefield, 1973–84).
RPCS   *Register of the Privy Council of Scotland,* third series, 1660–91, 16 vols., various editors (Edinburgh, 1908–80).
SRO   Scottish Record Office.

Because so many kirk sessions registers are now in local archives, we have not provided SRO references to them. The registers can all be traced via the SRO, and as we have provided the month and year in our quotations and allusions, the relevant volumes can easily be located.

Introduction

Western societies have social rules that sex and childbearing should be confined within a formalised bond of marriage. Until recent times these rules were very strong, conflicting with and usually overriding powerful personal sexual impulses. People suspected of breaking them would provoke a social response, scandalised gossip at the least. Suspicion and gossip are ephemeral, but the birth of a child outside wedlock is the plainest possible evidence of rule breaking, and the community would be bound to react. Both the circumstances leading to that birth, and the nature of the reaction, are of interest to the historian.

Our original aim in this study was to measure illegitimacy in Scotland in the seventeenth and eighteenth centuries. We were particularly interested in variations over time, in a 120 year period of social and economic change. We also wanted to look at regional patterns, in a country where geography has preserved cultural and linguistic subgroups from each other and from English influence, yet which has also cohered around a remarkable homogeneity of religious belief, law, education and ethics. It was the excellent records of the kirk sessions – the parish church disciplinary courts – that made such a study feasible. But we quickly realised that our original aim was too narrow, and that a much broader study could, and should, be conducted.

First we had to understand the mental and moral world in which these illegitimate births occurred, and so this book begins by outlining the theology which sustained church discipline, and the court structure which administered it. We then had to review (Chapter 2) the changing economic and social setting, because of its profound links with sexuality and fertility. For instance, marriage was supposed to be restricted to those who could afford to support a family, and servant girls were not free to marry but could fall prey to the sexual advances of their masters. In any case what did it mean to be married, in law or in public opinion, in a country whose border town Gretna is synonymous with ideas, customs and myths around marriage quite different from England's? Some marriages were irregularly contracted yet legally sound, and the births legitimate, whereas other unions were beyond the pale; so only when we had clarified the regular and irregular state of affairs (Chapters 3 and 4) and dispelled some myths could we study those births deemed illegitimate (Chapter 5). So comprehensive proved the kirk sessions records that we often learnt how, when and why these pregnancies occurred, and how the individuals responded to them and to being confronted by authority (Chapters 6 and 7). We found a fascinating range of deviant behaviour, from 'anticipating the marriage' to seduction, adultery and outright rape; and of responses from contrition and official forgiveness to defiance, flight, and excommunication from Church and Christian society.

One reason for such comprehensive records is that the Scottish Church in the early modern period was engrossed by the sexual irregularities of its flock; indeed it seems

Girls in Trouble

at times to have thought of little else. It evinced extreme distaste for any show of physical intimacy between the sexes outwith marriage, and would penalise any such 'scandalous carriage' whenever it could not prove a graver offence of fornication. And although Scotland ceased to be a church-ruled society by around 1780, when our study ends, it did continue to have a keen sense of itself as a moral nation, and to be affronted by sexual lapses. This sense was reinforced by the moralistic flavour of nineteenth-century middle-class Britain, and by romantic notions of the virtues of rural life as opposed to the sinful, teeming cities. With pride the Scot could contemplate Scottish education, Scottish poor law and other civic provisions, the pious peace of a Scottish Sunday; and the rest of the world (not least a Balmoralistic royalty) tended to share this image of a chaste and godly land. But then some inconvenient facts came to light.

Those facts emerged after the setting up of civil registration for Scotland in 1855 and the Census of 1861. What they revealed was an overall illegitimacy ratio of 9.4 per cent; for urban areas it was 9.2 per cent, and for rural areas 9.5 per cent. In the south-west, where presbyterianism was said to be particularly strong, it was over 13 per cent, and in some parishes it exceeded 30 per cent. England, by contrast, scored 6 to 7 per cent. There was some explaining to do.

Some of those explanations were technical – there are drawbacks to using ratios that will be discussed in Chapter 5 – but that did not obviate the problem of stark local variations. Why, for instance, was a teenage girl in Banffshire twenty times more likely to have an illegitimate child than one in Ross and Cromarty? And what was to be done about it? Much effort was put into shepherding the errant population towards a chaster way of life, but with limited success, and marked regional variations in illegitimacy persisted well into the twentieth century. That was partly because of a distinctly one-sided definition of where the problem lay, and of what solutions were appropriate. The secular state was not prepared to adopt policies which challenged property rights, or obliged farmers to make suitable provision for their married workers. The church increasingly saw moral deviance as located in those who fell pregnant, not in those who impregnated. Illegitimacy in Scotland reflected a confluence of economic, social and biological forces, but it was the girls who were in trouble.

Our own interest in this area was prompted by (and is in some senses a continuation of) this very long-standing concern with the sexuality and social control of the people of Scotland. These high overall ratios and marked regional variations: how far back did they go? Did they pre-date the onset of capitalised agriculture, and the great move from the land to the towns? Did illegitimacy rise in isolation, or in parallel with overall and legitimate fertility? What changes took place in the rules about illegitimacy and other sexual behaviours, and what theories might we put to the test?

Scottish demography became a much more exact science after 1855 when legislation created a system of civil registration of births, deaths and marriages. The equivalent English system was set up earlier, in 1838, and before that there had been a much more complete system of parish registration. In Scotland, despite legislation of the early seventeenth century, many of the Old Parish Registers (OPRs) were irregularly kept. By contrast, Scottish kirk sessions were rigorous in documenting any pregnancy in an unmarried woman, and enough of their registers survive to be sure of drawing a representative picture. Several hundred parishes have left carefully

Introduction

kept registers for the eighteenth century, and over 200 survive from the late seventeenth century. For strong doctrinal reasons (set out in Chapter 1), Scottish church discipline had to be comprehensive and systematic, else one's very salvation was in doubt, and there was regular inspection of the records by the higher church authorities. Above all, there was an astonishingly effective system of church detective work and community support. Offenders could expect to be detected and summonsed, could not blithely ignore the church courts, and found it very difficult to flee beyond their justice. None of this would be true of England in that period; only the Isle of Man comes anywhere near.

The limits to our study reflect the limits to our confidence in this material. Before 1660 there were too many disturbances to civic order: the wars against England, participation in the English Civil War, civil war within Scotland, military conquest by England. These disturbances continued well beyond 1660 in some districts, which to that extent have been excluded from study. By 1780 the system of church discipline was breaking down, so our study ends there. This is a great shame because we are forced to break off just as Scotland was encountering the transformation of its agriculture, and its industrial revolution. In one crucial respect however we made a wrong assumption about the kirk sessions. We assumed that the Church could never enforce discipline in the mushrooming cities, and only then discovered that it tried hard, and left good records. A second research study was put in hand once we realised this, the results of which appear in a companion book to this one, *Sin in the City*.

For the research described in the present book, of the 900 or so parishes in early modern Scotland we picked 78 for detailed analysis, on three criteria. First, there should be no obvious problem of quality of the surviving records. Second, they should cover a reasonable time span; indeed some parishes cover over 100 years with few or no breaks, while individual ministers lived and died, and world events marched on around them. Third, they should take in the main regions of Scotland, with enough parishes and enough of a population base in each regional subsample to ensure a representative picture. This is essential, as single parishes could be highly idiosyncratic in either the frequency of illegitimacy or other deviance, or in the way society responded to it.

That, alas, ruled out three regions: the Northern Isles and the Western Isles, through lack of enough early material, and the Borders because of massive depopulation during the eighteenth century (we did however study its experience of irregular marriage, which was made easy by its nearness to England). Inevitably, we left out some counties, such as Angus, Mearns (Kincardineshire) and Lanarkshire, where we decided that the adjacent regions were near enough in character. And, as explained earlier, the cities were here ignored.

We grouped the 78 parishes into five regions from south of the Highland line (Dumbarton to Stonehaven) and five from the north. In the south: the Lothians, conspicuous throughout our period for relatively prosperous farming, a pattern of large landowning units and closeness to central government. Fife was also near to government but agriculturally poor, isolated by the Firth of Forth to the south and the Tay to the north, and with important industries such as mining, salt works and fisheries. The Central Lowlands of Stirlingshire and southern Perthshire were prosperous in farming but experienced both the advantages and disadvantages of being adjacent to the Highlands. Ayrshire in the west had an economy based on good farm lands, ports and (later) coal and salt. Finally Dumfries and Galloway in the south-west, an area of decaying ports, hilly terrain and mild climate. Galloway had very high illegitimacy in the nineteenth century, a very long tradition of separate laws, and in the seventeenth century was notoriously resistant to the ecclesiastical policy of the Crown.

In the north: the north-east corner of Moray, Banffshire and Nairnshire was economically a mixed area, a coastal string of ports backed by a narrow strip of rich farm land with a mild climate, and giving way to a highland belt. (This was another area to show high illegitimacy in the late nineteenth century.) Aberdeenshire was the heart of agriculture and, like the north-east, had long favoured the Episcopal Church and included notable enclaves of Roman Catholicism. Caithness, a lowland economy north of the Highlands, was predominately English-speaking as early as the eighteenth century, but its culture sprang from the Norse. Finally there were two highland regions, the western Highlands, and the central and eastern. These were Gaelic-speaking areas in which, at the beginning of our period, the government had only limited ability to make its wishes felt.

These regional groupings would, we trust, look obvious not only to a modern Scot, but to the people of our period 1660–1780. Their boundaries are often sharp, reflecting a geographic barrier or a linguistic change. We appreciate that we may have missed interesting features in the counties not studied. Nevertheless we feel confident that a picture of Scotland drawn from these 78 parishes is a fair one. It is also much more complete than those drawn for other countries where illegitimacy in this period has been studied.

1

The Scottish Church

After 1560 the prevailing ethic of post-Reformation Scotland, and the formal system of social control, were based on Calvinist dogma. Calvinism held to the sinfulness of man, and the uselessness of any form of good works for the achievement of salvation. Its central feature was the total gulf between God and man. God was almighty and the creator of the world: man, his creation, was corrupted in all his activities by the taint of original sin. There could be no merit or virtue in man except that attributed to him by God, though God was capable of working through human actions for His own ends. Everything that had happened, or would in future time happen, was known by and determined by God; including whether each individual would be saved or damned ('predestination').

Indeed, in 'supralapsarian' theology, which took hold in the early seventeenth century, the division of mankind into the 'elect', those to whom God had allotted salvation, and the 'reprobate', destined to damnation, had been made before the Fall. This doctrine required the arguing away or ignoring of the New Testament teaching that Christ died to save all men from sin, and, at face value, it would make pointless any organised church on earth. Calvin nevertheless put great stress on the organisation of the Church and its relationship to secular powers. His follower, John Knox, who put his stamp on Scotland's Reformation, stressed even further the importance of the individual congregation. Within the congregation the sacrament of Holy Communion held a central place, for it celebrated communion with God/Christ, with the Church, and with one's fellow Christians. The priest or minister, who alone could administer this sacrament, had great prestige, enhanced by his exclusive duty of also preaching the Word, that is of expounding doctrine.

Only one other sacrament was recognised, that of baptism, but this, it was expressly stated in the Confession of Faith, was not necessary for salvation.[1] The sacraments were the sign and seal of membership of the Christian church. Justification, that is the attribution of righteousness by God, was by faith alone, and was not linked to any action on the part of the justified. This did not mean that those who assented to the dogmas of the Church were necessarily among those to be saved.

That all man's faculties and actions were corrupted by sin did not mean that all men were equally sinful. Those convinced that they were members of the elect (and assurance of this, vouchsafed by God, was an essential, and highly convenient, feature of such membership), were expected to show this in their daily life by abstaining from gross sins and by repentance after sinning. Calvinism thus called on all Christians not only to hold the right beliefs but also to keep the commandments and the moral laws, to hope that they would gain assurance, and in this way to further God's will.

As a means of securing and encouraging the believers in acting in accordance with God's commands there developed covenant theology. This postulated the covenant of grace, an agreement between Christ and his flock by which redemption was promised to the elect. The elect would receive the gift of the Holy Ghost and be sustained in faith by the Church and the sacraments. This theology tied election to the fulfilment of God's will, not to membership of the Church, which would counter any suggestion that the assured could ignore the commandments. In Scotland covenant theology led to formal renewals of the National Confession of Faith, and subscription to it. Since the original protestant confession of 1560 declared that a godly discipline was one of the signs of the true Church, the renewal of the confession reaffirmed the necessity of membership of the Church and subjection to its rules. The true Church was the body of the elect: the Confession defined the Church as a 'company and multitude of men chosen by God', so a congregation could not consider itself part of this company unless it sustained discipline. The system of regular discipline enforced by the church courts in Scotland in the early modern period was therefore an essential part of the affirmation by the community of its membership of the elect. If they did not enforce Christian discipline, their very salvation was in doubt.[2]

There was a further reason for the enforcement of discipline which extended beyond Calvinism to all Christian denominations. God was seen as likely to intervene directly in human affairs: this did not contradict the concept of predestination, for God had many ways of achieving his aims. His intervention was likely if He was affronted by the behaviour of mankind, and would lead to chastisement. In other words, a nation which tolerated sinful behaviour, and let it proliferate, would deserve to suffer disaster: plagues, famines, riots, rebellions and the like. Morality was therefore an important element of national security. The Scottish Church reflected this view not only in sermons from all colours of ecclesiastical opinion during the 1745 Jacobite rising,[3] but also by the general habit of imposing a day of fasting and humiliation whenever the physical or political climate turned harsh.

All individuals were expected to make a positive adherence to the Church: i.e. to understand its theology, to obey its rules and to aim all the time at a godly life, for to fail to do so was to declare oneself reprobate. But these ideas were accepted by a society highly unequal in wealth and authority. Christianity did not make all men equal, still less make women equal to men. When a congregation affirmed its covenant, very noticeably in the National Covenant of 1638, the affirmation was by men only. Naturally landowners expected those of lesser rank to be under their authority. In June 1656 the laird of Brodie had this debate with his sister:

> She said, thes that should be heirs of glori with us, we oght not to compt the less of them for outward thing. I replied, Heirs of glori did not exeem them from al civil duties and subjection on earth. He might have more grace then I, and sit above me in heaven, that wer not to goe befor me, nay, nor be considerd besid me on earth.

Landowner authority did not confine itself to worldly matters. In 1654 the males of this family had renewed their covenants by pledging their souls and bodies, lands and houses, wives, children and servants to God.[4] Their women folk confirmed this pledge: the assent of the servants seems to have been taken for granted.

Reformation Scotland was a country with little real power in the hands of the central authority, the Crown. In many areas great feudatories exercised the functions of government, in the form of justice and military authority; nominally as delegates of the monarch, but in practice near to independence. Such great lords also intercepted parts of the royal revenue. The Crown had, in many areas, no officials directly responsible to it alone. So by establishing a hierarchy of church courts and by settling ministers responsible to these courts in the parishes, the Church enjoyed a far more effective system of government than the State. Its ministers were professionally trained, and held by a professional ethos, whereas agents of the Crown, such as Justices of the Peace or Commissioners of Supply, were qualified by being landowners, and had the ethics of owners of inherited property. Only gradually did they exempt themselves from the dominance of the great feudatories. By the mid-seventeenth century most parishes had a minister of religion, and a kirk session, a permanent committee made up of minister and elders. Elders were elected by the existing session members. Elders were men of local note or distinction, but the distinction did not have to be great, for the session usually selected at least one elder from every settlement in the parish. In the seventeenth century many of the elders were unable to read, but by the mid-eighteenth century, the school system these men had helped to create meant that such a disability was rare. Some of the elders were landowners, but the session needed more elders than the landowning class could provide, and tenants and merchants supplied these. In the towns the sessions drew on merchants, craftsmen and members of the professions.

From soon after the Reformation, in some cases even before it was politically achieved, the structure of the Church's government was being built up. By the early seventeenth century it was agreed that ministers were nominally equal in status and function, even though the Crown had planted an episcopal structure on the Church. There was a hierarchy of church courts, the kirk session for parish business, above it the presbytery, then the synod, with the General Assembly, a meeting ground for the whole Church and the source of ecclesiastical legislation, at the top.[5]

The court above the kirk session was the presbytery, and this was the focus of Church authority under the presbyterian system. It was the presbyteries that raised topics for discussion by the General Assembly, and decided which parishes should send representatives there. (Indeed, after 1697 proposals and rulings could not be made in the General Assembly until they had been referred to all the presbyteries.) Presbyteries contained all the ministers within their areas. In the Restoration period the elders were not included in the membership of presbyteries, or of synods, but they were restored to these in 1689. However, in the eighteenth century they seldom attended. Travel was difficult and expensive, and neither the formal business of the meeting nor the informal network of contacts there would have motivated their attendance. Elders who did attend these courts were usually men of the upper class.

The presbytery also held a key position in the system of discipline, for the penalty of lesser excommunication, which cut an offender off from communion, was under its control. Lesser excommunication could, until 1712, lead to referral of an offender for imprisonment by the sheriff. Greater excommunication, which cut an offender off from all contact with anyone outside his household and prohibited movement away from the parish, was under the control of the bishop (after 1689 of the synod), but this was a sentence too drastic to be used except very occasionally.

In the episcopal period, that is before 1690, the induction of new ministers was by presbytery and bishop; after 1690 by presbytery alone, though in disputed cases the presbytery might be reinforced by outside ministers. Presbyteries heard candidates for the ministry go through their trials, appointed ministers when the rights of patrons had lapsed, and between 1690 and 1712 'cognosed', or arbitrated, in disputes when appointments were by heritors and elders but also to be approved by heads of households. They supervised the record-keeping of the kirk sessions (though their instructions on the detailed presentation of information were not always followed), provided some level of services during vacancies, put pressure, where necessary, on landowners to perform their duties in building and maintaining church, manse and school, and the conduct and doctrine of ministers, dealt with disciplinary cases which were beyond the competence of the session, and mediated in quarrels between landowners and their ministers.

There were over 900 parishes, and 62 presbyteries, in Scotland at the start of the eighteenth century. New units were continually carved out of older ones, or older units were combined, according to the sense of the General Assembly of religious, financial or administrative need, and so there can be no fixed number asserted for our period as a whole. Parishes usually had a population of between 600 and 3,000, and often covered a large geographical area; 80 square miles would be unremarkable. The population was normally not grouped in any nuclear village but was scattered in smaller settlements, farm towns, or wherever there was a stretch of good farm land. Parishes were even larger in the Highlands, where their limited number reflected the difficulty of recruiting enough ministers who spoke Gaelic. In the Lowlands a conscientious minister would get round all the settlements regularly in his annual catechising, but in the Highlands his contact was less, particularly where there were no roads. Even in the Lowlands the size of many parishes made it unlikely that all parishioners could attend church regularly. The system of elders meant, however, that all settlements were in touch with the kirk session.

A kirk session met as often as business required. That is, it might meet weekly or even more frequently; rarely did more than a month go by without a meeting. In some parishes, though, the meetings were sparser. Session business involved poor relief, and money might be doled out monthly, quarterly or even by the half year. It also arranged church repairs and purchase of equipment; it levied fees for the use of church equipment at funerals, organised the annual communion service, arranged collections for good causes commended by the higher courts, supervised the school, and looked after visiting ministers during vacancies. Higher courts, when they sent requests or recommendations to the kirk sessions, would check up later on what the session had done. Some session registers record the text of the weekly sermons. It is clear from the quality of surviving records that the members of sessions were conscientious men who took their duties seriously. A session could manage most business effectively without a resident and active minister for about six months, but if a vacancy or serious illness went on for longer the conduct of business would become disorganised. But on discipline matters, cases were sometimes left ready for action when a minister should be appointed, rather than dealt with by the elders without their moderator.

The presbytery was a committee small enough to be effective and, to make sure that it was effective, regular attendance by the ministers was insisted on. It met several times a year, often monthly in the summer. It had no fixed base, being able to vary its meeting from parish to parish. This meant that it normally met in one fairly central location, but visited different parishes at intervals, inspecting the records and equipment. Many ministers could walk or ride to and from the meeting within the day, but even where a longer absence was involved the presbyteries insisted on punctual attendance. As it was a meeting of ministers, it was the body where discipline of errant ministers would be initiated. Under episcopacy the moderator or chairman was appointed by the bishop, often for six months or more at a time, but later was elected by the presbytery.

Above the presbytery came the synod. A synod approximated in size to a medieval diocese. It met twice a year for two or three days, in spring and autumn, with a good deal of formality. Disciplinary matters generally came before the synod only if for some reason the lower courts were not working effectively, for instance in disturbed parts of the Highlands. To that extent the main role of synod was to reinforce the authority of lower courts, not to act as an arbiter in its own right. However, it could be influential in politics and local government, and perhaps for this reason elders were more regular attenders here than at presbytery. Synods were especially important before 1689, under episcopacy, since, with the refusal of the government to call the General Assembly, it was the highest level of church court. Inevitably rulings about discipline and worship had to be made, and were, by synods. Synods also usually appointed days of fasting and humiliation, called for subscriptions to good causes (not always religious), and played a part in the workings of local government.[6]

Synods continued to be important in the Highlands after 1689, because of the weakness of presbyteries and sessions there, and because the large parishes meant that the ministers needed more support and control than elsewhere. The lack of Gaelic-speaking presbyterian ministers led to the synods pursuing a policy over selection very different from that of the General Assembly, and to the retention of many episcopal ministers in this area. A court of stature was also needed for negotiation with powerful chiefs and for sustaining the parish clergy against the pressures of Catholicism. All this enhanced the political dimension of the Synod of Argyll and, later, that of Glenelg. After the defeat of the 1745 rising and the forced incorporation of the highland area into the normal government structure of Scotland this political aspect of the highland synods was reduced.[7]

The two intermediate courts were predominantly of clergy, and were places for the exercise of professional expertise. It is clear that the members of presbyteries were aware of the distinction of ranks and knew that it was not usually productive to quarrel with the landowning class.

At the top of the structure of church courts sat, when it was allowed to meet, the General Assembly. This met annually, in the early summer, but also had a committee, the Commission, which carried on business between meetings and which met three times a year. The General Session of Edinburgh was always represented, while representation of other parishes was rotated. The General Assembly was considered politically dangerous in the Restoration period, and though an Act was passed defining its membership, it was not called till 1689, when a highly unrepresentative presbyterian group claimed this status.[8] In spite of the continually changing nature of its membership the Assembly in the eighteenth century had a strong party structure, at first being divided between the episcopal and presbyterian camps, later between the so-called evangelical or popular party and the moderates. The Assembly did not normally hear disciplinary cases, except where ministers were accused of heresy or misbehaviour, but the Commission got involved in some when individuals appealed there against the decision of their presbytery.

The Scottish presbyterian system was basically an oligarchy, open to selected social groups. The activity of laymen was most conspicuous in the lowest and the highest courts, but the men so involved were of widely different rank and performed different functions. In the kirk session laymen were the greater part of the membership, and played a vital part in conducting the sessions' business, though they did not fill the post of moderator. Membership was for life, though an elder might take periods of retirement. It carried considerable responsibility, not only for making decisions but also for handling the parish's money. By contrast, the laymen who attended the General Assembly did so only occasionally, and had no political organisation in it. Assembly time was, for those selected by the presbyteries to attend, mainly an occasion for social life, but also, in the case of lawyers, an opportunity to pick up useful business.

The strength of this court structure must strike anyone who works in its records. The courts suffered no lapse by death. Regular record keeping was imposed by their superiors. A uniformity in policy permeated the whole system, unusual in a country with so much regional diversity as Scotland, for the meetings of the courts not only provided formal regulation and definitions, but also opportunities for the exchange of ideas about how to handle particular types of issue. The result was that a kirk session in Easter Ross would be making disciplinary decisions in much the same way as one in Wigtownshire. Occasional translation of a minister from one parish to another also helped to maintain uniformity. The courts of the Church had a great advantage over secular justice, in that they were worked free of charge by salaried people. If a woman brought a complaint against her husband to her session, or a session called on a man named as father of a bastard child to answer the accusation, no costs were incurred. Only when a member of the upper class was embarrassed by an allegation and wished to repel it with legal support would lawyers appear in these courts. The ministers lived on their stipends, and the officials of the court who called on people to appear and the clerks who kept the records received small salaries funded out of the church collections. It seems that the ministers paid for the cost of postal services to enquire about missing offenders and to check upon documentation submitted to the session.

Thus, even by the early seventeenth century the Church was an institution equipped with a far more modern system of government than the State, so it is not surprising that it got involved in matters of political and penal policy. Religion was, after all, an important political issue: nobody could ignore this after the events of 1637–38 when aristocratic opponents to the policy of Charles I successfully fanned the popular hostility to the new Prayer Book into outright revolution. Ever since the Reformation the Church had seen major decisions on policy as within its sphere of influence. It assented to the idea of a separation of Church and State, but took this to mean that the Church governed itself whereas the Crown was merely the practical administrator of the wishes of God, which would, if necessary, be defined for it by the Church. So the early General Assemblies called for specific penalties on what they saw as sins, and expected these to be passed into legislation and imposed by the State. An example of this is the post-Reformation view that death should be the penalty for adultery, a view which the Crown, conscious of the sexual failings of many of the aristocracy, was not prepared to enact.[10] The Church felt at liberty to denounce the behaviour of the great, including the monarch himself, either in general terms as lacking in Christian zeal, or for particular shortcomings, and to close its eyes to moral failures by its allies.

All moral failures were, in its eyes, its sphere of action, but it also recognised that God would work in mysterious ways and by dubious instruments. It also saw immoral acts as inherently objectionable to God, and was not particularly concerned over the mental state and the intentions of the offender, or the social desirability of penalties. For instance, it was persistently hostile to the policy of compensation for murder. The Crown used this policy in the early seventeenth century in order to end feuds, but the Church objected to the imposing of different penalties for the same offence on different ranks. It was the Church's view which prevailed eventually.[11]

The Church had, of necessity, to carry out functions of government which, in the modern world, are regarded as secular. Until the mid-nineteenth century it was in charge of education and poor relief. The latter role came from the incoherence and inefficiency of such lay local government as existed in the seventeenth century. When we find a synod promoting a secular cause, such as the fund-raising for bridges or harbours, we can see the Church stepping into a gap in the lay State.

From 1661 to 1689 the Church of Scotland had not only a presbyterian system of government but also an episcopal one. The dioceses of the bishops were coterminous with the synods. Bishops had their own administrative staff. They were involved in the disciplining of ministers for misbehaviour or inadequate doctrinal conformity, acted as permanent moderators of synods, might associate with presbyteries for particular activities, and either appointed or themselves were moderators.[12] But they seem to have had little effect at parish level. The political pressures of this period in Scotland and the waywardness of Crown policy caused the episcopate to become closely associated with the monarchy. Bishops had no strong territorial base, and were not linked to the major landowners. So, when the direct Stewart line was forced out in the Revolution of 1688–89 the episcopate could not accept the intrusion of William III and Mary as monarchs, and became 'Jacobite'. The new monarchy, with no core of bishops on its side, was forced to allow the establishment of a totally presbyterian system. The self-selected General Assembly, made up entirely of ministers untainted by the Restoration church system, ruthlessly purged over two-thirds of the ministry over the next few years and intruded its own candidates into the parishes so vacated.

This drastic change in the officiating ministry clearly impacted upon the Church at parish level. In some parishes, mostly in the north-east, where it was difficult for the Assembly to get in its candidates because of popular support for the existing men, there were riots and disturbances; in some parishes almost a state of organised disruption for many years.[13] Some of the new ministers were anxious to display zeal. In Cramond, Midlothian, for instance, the new minister's arrival is shown in a surge of prosecutions for Sabbath breach. But the discipline of sex offences does not seem to have been affected by discontinuity and disturbance. The elders might postpone action if there was a vacancy, until a new minister had been installed. But the resulting surge in cases gives a distorted picture of normal parish life, and partly for this reason this study has omitted years when there was clearly a break in kirk session business. But there was no change in the general policy regarding such cases. The Episcopalian Church, as it came to be called, and the Presbyterian agreed on doctrine and discipline, and carried on the same policy through the Revolution.

Union with England in 1707 brought considerable changes in secular justice, but seems to have had little direct effect on the Church. Ministers continued to treat England as a foreign country, and the receipt of English ministrations for marriage or baptism as a church offence. But the ensuing Toleration Act of 1712 left its mark on the Scottish system of church courts. By this Act the Episcopalian Church was allowed to hold its own services and use its own service book, so that while the established Church claimed jurisdiction over all parish residents, it could hardly exercise discipline over episcopalians without the co-operation of episcopal clergy. After the 1715 Jacobite rising, in which the episcopal clergy was clearly shown as disaffected to the government, services in meeting houses were made legally dependent on the minister having taken the oaths of allegiance and assurance, and this restricted the level of official toleration promised by the Toleration Act. The Act also removed the right of the Church to call on the sheriff to imprison those under excommunication, but this had been so rarely invoked that it was not of importance.

There were, from 1689 and even before, some minor sects, such as the Quakers, and there was also a small, scattered organisation of covenanters, who were not prepared to follow the main body of covenanting opinion into the Presbyterian Church, but dissent within protestantism played a very small role in early eighteenth-century Scotland. The Original Secession of 1733 was a small and local affair of an extremely scrupulous and puritanical group. But the Relief Church, which came into existence in the 1750s, was wider in its support, and ready to accept a wide range of opinion. It is thus only in the 1760s that dissent became significant, and involved a considerable minority of the people in communions outwith the establishment.[14]

The Church's system of government underwent remarkably little change in the period of this study. The disappearance of episcopacy left the system working in practice much as before. More important was the simultaneous re-establishment of the General Assembly, which gradually became representative of the Church as a whole, and which, by its existence, reduced the importance of the synods. The other change of long-term significance was the break in presbyterian unity, and the consequent springing up of dissenting communions. The civil government of Scotland experienced much greater changes. It expanded not only by institutional change but also by a general increase in efficacy and authority. The new central criminal court, the Court of Justiciary, is important in this connection, and so is the creation, in the Commissioners of Supply, of a mechanism for local valuation and taxation.[15]

But the major change in civil government was the enhanced authority of the State from the Restoration period. In the period of the Great Rebellion the Scottish aristocracy were politically defeated by the Church and shown as dispensable in government. Eventually the country had been conquered by England. English success in suppressing a major rising in the Highlands had shown that even in that area armies from the low country could penetrate and exert control. All these events showed that no area of Scotland was immune from control, and that Scotland could not afford to quarrel with England. In the Restoration the aristocracy had been restored along with the monarchy, but even when noblemen had cleared their estates of the debts produced by the wars and by fines, the lessons of the Rebellion period were not lost. Even the mightiest men in the land recognised that a moderate degree of co-operation with central government and obedience to the law were essential for survival. Though large territorial franchises continued to exist until the 1740s, and so excluded parts of the country from the authority of the Crown's courts, law and order had become firmly established in the Lowlands. In the Highlands, though endemic warfare continued until the 1690s, it was on a much smaller scale than in the past.

1: The Scottish Church

Highland chiefs found it necessary to maintain some sort of contact with the central government, and for this reason had to restrain some of their more lawless clansmen.[16]

Union with England in 1707 provided a further strength for the forces of order. It led to the enhancement of the functions of the central courts, and to their encroachment into the areas of the franchises.[17] The membership of the Court of Session gradually shifted from appointments simply by political patronage to one of patronage modified by the recognition of professional ability. This change led to the great age of the development of Scots law and of authoritative works on it. Some of this law looks like the improvisation of judges, prompted by the interests and ethos of landed society, but these features did not damage their overall authority.

The judges and advocates who worked the legal system were gentry, that is they were owners of moderate sized estates. The same section of society provided the sheriffs, Justices of the Peace and Commissioners of Supply. Whereas in the seventeenth century this section of society had been overshadowed and bullied by the great lords, it now became a secure and independent layer in society. The aristocracy, already tamed by the Great Rebellion, now was deflected by the allure of London.[18] These changes meant that the government of Scotland in the eighteenth century approximated closely to that of England in lay matters, with local administration and justice in the hands of the gentry. The difference between them was that in Scotland the lay system provided only part of the arrangements for social control, the other part being the church courts. Until the mid-eighteenth century there were also baron courts, in which farming disputes were settled and the landowners' orders and interests promoted.

The combined systems of authority, ecclesiastical and lay, and the tenurial system, all meant that the population of Scotland was held to obedience by a strong and interlaced set of bonds.[19] There is no reason for thinking that this was distasteful to those controlled by it. Amongst the groups below gentry level some had much greater liberty than others: for instance miners, nominally serfs, had an effective trade union system which enabled them to resist pressure by the mineowners to increase output.[20] There were also occasions in the year when disorder or misrule were accepted. Saints days were supposed to have disappeared at the Reformation, but New Year replaced Christmas as a festival and became an occasion for heavy drinking, and Shrove Tuesday was observed with orgiastic enthusiasm. Other uproarious days were the fairs, particularly the hiring fairs, and of course weddings. But in spite of these occasions for breach of order, or perhaps because of them, it seems that most people of both sexes accepted the systems of control under which they lived, and actively co-operated with that of the Church. The abolition of the sanction of imprisonment by the sheriff for those incurring lesser excommunication in 1712 had no effect on the level of obedience to the courts of the Church.

Such effective church discipline by the Scottish Kirk marks that country out from the rest of the British Isles in the eighteenth century. The English reformed churches aimed at this sort of discipline, but none was remotely as successful as the Scottish Church in the seventeenth century, even less so in the eighteenth. For instance, neither seventeenth-century Wiltshire, nor Cromwellian Somerset, could effectively discipline sexual misconduct, as it was too easy for offenders to move away and be lost sight of.[21] From the Isle of Man flight was less easy, and Anglican discipline persisted into the mid-eighteenth century, but penalties were mild and that for fornication was waived if the couple subsequently married.[22]

Clearly the efficacy of any system of discipline depends on its comprehensiveness. In England the refusal by the gentry to be subject to control or censure by the Church was one reason for the weakness of discipline even in the early seventeenth century. Later the proliferation of dissent meant that the Established Church could not be seen, and did not see itself, as responsible for the entire populace. Yet in the early seventeenth century illegitimacy in England appears to have been low. Though the nadir of the illegitimacy ratio was achieved at a time when not all births were being registered (for there was widespread objection to the civil registration imposed by the Commonwealth government), the levels calculated for other decades are still strikingly low, and the number of parishes used as a base is large. Before the Civil War the material comes from a period when the unity of the Church had not been seriously fractured.[23]

The research in England has, in some cases, discovered the illegitimacies not recorded in the parish register by other means, e.g. burial registers. Parish registration also misses children dying unbaptised, and it is likely that in the seventeenth and early eighteenth centuries illegitimate children suffered higher perinatal mortality than those born within wedlock, as in later centuries. Parish clerks may have failed to enter some children as illegitimates, but the trend of the figures is remarkably consistent, suggesting that the level of omission was not great. The law imposing parish registration was effective in England and the age of baptism in the seventeenth century very low.[24] Even though the Church had a less effective discipline over its ministers than had the Scottish Church, and ministers were allowed a certain amount of non-residence and plurality, which might prevent them being fully familiar with their parishioners, the English figures are a convincingly stable understatement of the level of illegitimacy.

In Scotland parish registration, though ordered in 1616 for baptisms and burials, was, as in many other areas of statutory regulation, effectively optional. A typical parish was Tranent, East Lothian, where, with all deliberate speed, a register of burials was opened only in 1753, and kept for less than thirty years.[25] There was no strong pressure to get children to the font quickly after birth since baptism was not necessary for salvation.

English parish recording might miss some cases of illegitimacy, but the parish ratepayers were concerned not be saddled with the support of bastards. The English Poor Law led to a secular motive for the repression of unmarried sexual activity, and also meant that illegitimate births were likely to be noted in other places than the parish register. This fact, combined with the proliferation of local record keeping and the smallness of many English parishes, means that more information about the social setting of illegitimacy cases can often be elicited for England than is possible for Scotland. Even so, we agree with Keith Wrightson (referring to the Interregnum but of more general relevance) that there was 'no simple pattern of moral regulation'.[26] The established Church in England never had the disciplinary authority that distinguished the Church of Scotland.

The Scottish system of control of individuals by the Church was not only much more effective than the English, it also extended for a longer time, continuing through the third quarter of the eighteenth century, only to end abruptly after that. There were not the pockets of resistant dissent comparable to those in seventeenth-century England.

1: The Scottish Church

Doctrinal and ecclesiastical unity meant that the most likely blocks to the mechanisms of control would come from laziness or inefficiency rather than from basic disagreement, and the higher courts of the Church did their best to prevent such faults persisting. Men and women were not, for much of our period, allowed to move from one parish to another without a certificate of good behaviour, a 'testificat', from their past parish, and these documents were not issued as a matter of course. Because of this practice, one of the main reasons for the ineffectiveness of moral discipline in England, the disappearance to some other area of the offender, did not apply in Scotland. The kirk session receiving a testificat would, through the minister, examine it carefully, as it would certificates of marriage from outwith the parish. If there were any doubts about authenticity, the documentation would be checked. Errors in terminology or handwriting would be perceived, and the minister would then write to the minister of the parish from which it was supposed to have emanated, and enquire about its authenticity. In the case of parishes within the same presbytery, the information could easily be obtained at the next meeting of the presbytery, otherwise the post would be used. Enquiries about offenders who had fled to one of the cities would often elicit accurate information as to where they were. Sessions even advertised in newspapers for information about missing suspects. The handwriting of those people of whom the Church disapproved, who made an income by selling irregular marriages, was well known to many sessions. Study of kirk session registers sometimes gives the impression that the detective system of the Kirk was an important element in the financial success of the postal service.

Offenders could thus be traced so long as they were within the area of effective church organisation. But fugitives might go further than this. In central and northern Scotland people might run away to the Highlands, though they usually did not stay there long. In the south-east they might go to the Netherlands, in the Border area to England, in Galloway to Ulster. Such flight certainly put people beyond the authority of the Kirk, but it might place a heavy strain on them, and it did not expunge the record. Return after many years would lead to the re-opening of the enquiry.

The Kirk treated England as a foreign country. Claims of marriage or baptism there would be treated with considerable scepticism, but were not ignored: support and proof would be asked for. The Scottish Kirk had a low opinion of Anglican discipline and was sceptical of claims of marriage by English divines, which, in the absence in England of a system of 'testificats' might not be easy to check.

There were still groups that the Church in Scotland could not fully control. At the head of these came the landowning class. Only for a brief period after the political change of 1649 was the Church in a position to extend discipline to such people. A session would, however, note a claim that paternity of a child was attributed to a landowner, though sometimes it was unreasonably anxious to preserve the reputation of such a man (see Chapter 7), and if the accusation was sustained and given support the session would at least enquire of the landowner if he agreed in its truth. Discipline could not be brought to bear on such men, but they might make penitential payment to the parish's poor fund. Discipline also could not be enforced upon the servants of the upper class.

Another group enjoying immunity was the army. Soldiers were not under the discipline of the parish, though if named, they might agree to meet with members of the session and give an account of their actions. Sometimes the military authority would co-operate with a session in helping a girl to get married to her lover, but by contrast some superior officers prevented their men marrying. An officer could refuse a man a certificate that he was not married, and almost force a soldier into an extra-marital liaison. For the most part, when it was alleged that a soldier was the father of an illegitimate child all that a session could do was to record the statement and make the girl do her penance.

A final area of doubt may remain, the question of whether all the people were firmly attached to one or another parish. Andrew Fletcher of Saltoun claimed in 1698 that in normal times 100,000 people in Scotland were vagrants living wild in the hills, spurning Christian ordinances, and that in times of dearth the number went up to 200,000. 'In all time,' he wrote, 'there have been about 100,000 of them Vagabond who have lived without any regard or subjection either to the Laws of the Land, or even those of God and Nature.' And he accused these people of incest, murder and coercive begging. 'In years of Plenty many thousands of these meet together in the Mountains, where they feast and riot for many days. At country Weddings, Burials and other the like publick occasions they are to be seen both Men and Women perpetually drunk.'[27]

We have studied 225 KSRs for the period, the 1690s, when this was written, a time of severe food shortage, and could not find a scrap of evidence for such a horde of outlaws. The registers do show that more people than usual were on the roads looking for some form of support in those years of scarcity. Fletcher reached his figures from class prejudice multiplied by total innumeracy, plus a few extra noughts on the end for colour and emphasis. He was experiencing a type of 'moral panic'; the reaction of settled and propertied rural society to the existence of small numbers of mobile people who do not conform to their norms. A characteristic of this hostility is to accuse the deviant population of sexual offences, living on welfare and evading honest work.

Certainly there were people living by travelling, but these 'vagrants' were not just the rejects of the economy. They included the valuable group of chapmen (roving pedlars and storytellers) and their families, old women collecting rags for the newly started paper industry, families migrating to and from England, demobilised and injured soldiers, and, particularly in the 1690s, dispossessed episcopal ministers and their families.[28] But such people appear in the records of almsgiving by the kirk sessions only in ones or twos. At communions and at 'publick occasions', where indiscriminate almsgiving was a common practice, people would flock in from neighbouring parishes, but these were not permanent vagrants, merely poor people keen to pick up small sums. The vagrancy element was not large, and many of the people who occur occasionally as 'stranger beggars' had firm parochial settlements and indulged in the various vices listed by Fletcher no more than anyone else.

The effectiveness of the parochial system was therefore strong, though in Galloway in the later seventeenth century there was a widespread repudiation of the ministry of the established Church, and in parts of the Highlands chronic disorder sometimes made it impossible for ministers to reside in their parishes; more often, they were unable to do parish visiting. Occasionally there are gaps in the session record. Sometimes during a vacancy in the ministry the slips of paper on which records were kept before they were inserted in the session register became confused or duplicated. But since each of our illegitimacy cases would normally appear in the register at least half a dozen times, starting with the allegation that an unmarried girl was pregnant, recording her statements and those of her named associate, their confessions when and if made, and ending with at least three recorded appearances in church by both, an occasional lapse does not prevent cases being noted. There might also be requests to have the child baptised.

More serious offences produced even more paper work, since the number of appearances escalated: whereas the sentence was three appearances for simple fornication, it was six for a 'relapse', that is a second offence, 26 for 'trilapse' or for adultery, 39 for 'quadrilapse' or relapse in adultery, and a whole year for incest.[29] These appearances were supposed to be made in sackcloth: a fine on each partner of ten pound Scots (16 shillings and eightpence sterling) was also exacted, though sometimes waived in cases of poverty. The literal minded approach to sin and to God's wrath imposed these high levels of penalty, without considering whether 39 appearances on the penitential pillar might not be counter-productive in terms of true penitence. Our research project has depended on the almost automatic insistence on the penalties and on the careful recording of every stage in the investigation. The outstanding quality of the record has enabled us to quantify illegitimacy, and to relate it to other forms of rule-breaking. In this record there can also be heard the response of people, including the accused, to the prospect of a birth out of wedlock. Whereas there is, for eighteenth-century England, a lack of information on the views of the lower orders on sexual matters,[30] Scotland has some examples of their voices.

Our study begins in 1660, by which time the presbyterian court system in the Church was well established, and the planting of ministers even in the remoter areas had made considerable progress. Apart from areas of surviving Roman Catholicism, which the Church frequently inquired into and for which the adherents were listed, and in spite of the survival of pagan rites in some areas, the Church had by 1660 achieved a near monopoly of religious organisation in Scotland, an effective government, a trained ministry and a generally accepted theology.[31] We did not try to take the study before 1660, for the combined effects of revolution, war and conquest made it likely that for some of the years before that date the system of church government was unlikely to be working smoothly. As a sample of this there is the gap in the kirk session register for Yester parish over the period covering the battle of Dunbar, followed by the note, 'No session was kept in our church betwixt the 22 of July 1650 and the 3 of August 1651 because of our troubles and absence of our minister.' We stopped the study in 1780 because of the obvious sudden deterioration in the system of church discipline. Possible reasons for this are discussed in Chapter 2. It is enough here to say that the change is unmistakable in most session registers at some point in the 1770s.

Notes

1 W.C. Dickinson (ed.), *John Knox's History of the Reformation in Scotland* (Edinburgh, 1949), vol. 2, Appendix 6.
2 We are grateful to Professor R.H. Campbell for our understanding of the doctrinal significance of discipline.
3 Richard B. Sher, *Church and University in the Scottish Enlightenment* (Edinburgh, 1985), pp. 43–4.
4 David Laing (ed.), *Diary of Alexander Brodie of Brodie MDCLII–MDCLIX and his son James Brodie of Brodie MDCLXXI–MDCLXXXV* (Spalding Club, Aberdeen, 1863),

Girls in Trouble

pp. 113, 180.
5   W.R. Foster, *The Church before the Covenants* (Edinburgh, 1975), Chs. 4–6.
6   W.R. Foster, *Bishop and Presbytery* (London, 1958), Ch. 4; G.D. Henderson, *Religious Life in Seventeenth-Century Scotland* (Cambridge, 1937), Ch. 7.
7   James Kirk (ed.), *The Records of the Synod of Lothian and Tweeddale* (Stair Society, Edinburgh, 1977), pp. ix–xxix; W. Ferguson, 'The Problems of the Established Church in the Western Highlands and Islands in the Eighteenth Century', *Records of the Scottish Church History Society 17* (1970), pp. 15–31.
8   A.L. Drummond and J. Bulloch, *The Scottish Church 1688–1843* (Edinburgh, 1973), Ch. 1.
9   Since the input to Assembly business came from the presbyteries, the impact of the laity was often of a negative kind, preventing outbursts of clericalism, but the lay membership was the mechanism by which the small moderate party maintained dominance in the late eighteenth century. Sher, *Church and University*, pp. 124–8.
10 J.R. Hardy, 'The attitudes of Church and State in Scotland to Sex and Marriage, 1560–1707' (unpublished M.Phil. thesis, Edinburgh University, 1978).
11 Jenny Wormald, 'Bloodfeud, Kindred and Government in early modern Scotland', *Past and Present 87* (1980), pp. 54–97.
12 Foster, *Bishop and Presbytery*, Ch. 3.
13 For instance the parish of Newtyle, Angus, seems from its KSR to have been the scene of near civil war for many years.
14 Drummond and Bulloch, *The Scottish Church*, Ch. 2.
15 Ann E. Whetstone, *Scottish county government in the eighteenth and nineteenth centuries* (Edinburgh, 1981), Ch. 3.
16 Paul Hopkins, *Glencoe and the end of the Highland War* (Edinburgh, 1986).
17 S.J. Davies, 'The courts and the Scottish legal system 1660–1747: the case of Stirlingshire', in V.A.C. Gatrell, Bruce Lenman and Geoffrey Parker (eds.), *Crime and the Law* (Cambridge, 1980), pp. 120–54.
18 J.S. Shaw, *The Management of Scottish Society* (Edinburgh, 1983), Ch. 1.
19 T.M. Devine, 'Unrest and Stability in Rural Ireland and Scotland, 1760–1840', in Rosalind Mitchison and Peter Roebuck (eds.), *Economy and Society in Scotland and Ireland, 1500–1939* (Edinburgh, 1988), pp. 126–39.
20 Christopher A. Whatley, 'The Fettering Bonds of Brotherhood: Combination and Labour Relations in the Scottish Coal Mining Industry, 1690–1775', *Social History* xii (1987), pp. 139–54.
21 M.J. Ingram, 'Church courts and neighbourhood: aspects of social control in Wiltshire, 1600–1641' (unpublished D.Phil. thesis, Oxford University, 1976); G.R. Quaife, *Wanton Wenches and Wayward Wives* (London, 1978), Chs. 8 and 9.
22 E.H. Stenning, 'Manx Spiritual Laws', *Isle of Man Natural History and Antiquarian Society Proceedings v* (1942–56), p. 287.
23 The figures are based on parish registration: one study used the registers of 24 parishes, distributed across much of the country, another a registration and family reconstitution in eight mainly southern parishes. Peter Laslett and Karla Oosterveen, 'Long-term trends in bastardy in England', *Population Studies* xxvii (1973), pp. 255–86; Karla Oosterveen, Richard M. Smith and Susan Stewart, 'Family reconstitution and the study of bastardy: evidence from certain English parishes', in Peter Laslett, Karla Oosterveen and Richard M. Smith (eds.), *Bastardy and its Comparative History* (London, 1980), pp. 86–140.
24 E.A. Wrigley and R. Schofield, *The Population History of England* (London, 1981), p. 289.
25 SRO CH2/357/21. Rosalind Mitchison, 'Death in Tranent', *Transactions of the East Lothian Antiquarian and Field Naturalists' Society* xvi (1979), pp. 37–48.
26 K. Wrightson, 'The nadir of English illegitimacy in the seventeenth century', in Laslett, Oosterveen and Smith (eds.), *Bastardy and its Comparative History*, pp. 176–91.
27 *Two Discourses Concerning the Affairs of Scotland* (1698), Second Discourse, pp. 24–9.

1: The Scottish Church

28 Rosalind Mitchison, 'Who were the poor in eighteenth-century Scotland?', in Mitchison and Roebuck (eds.), *Economy and Society in Scotland and Ireland, 1500–1939*, pp. 140–8.
29 Hardy, 'The attitudes of Church and State', p. 416.
30 Lawrence Stone, *The Family, Sex and Marriage in England 1500–1800*, Ch. 12.
31 Martin Martin, *A description of the Western Isles of Scotland circa 1695* (London, 1703); W. McKay (ed.), *Extracts from the presbytery records of Inverness and Dingwall* (Scottish History Society, Edinburgh, 1896); G.D. Henderson, *Religious Life* (Cambridge, 1937).

2

The Changing Economic and Social Setting

In Kilmartin parish, in July 1693, Katrin McGillivhide 'was rebuked for her sin of uncleanness, for defiling her body and soul that should be the pure temple of the Holy Ghost'. In January 1761, Elizabeth Downie 'acknowledged her having had the misfortune to be got with child upon the Hill of Southfarthing'. Both these statements epitomise the periods in which they were uttered and indicate how greatly attitudes – on the part of both Church and people – changed in the course of our period. The aim of this chapter is to chart the changes that took place and explain why they happened.

The years between those two unmarried pregnancies saw great changes in the economy, society and governing institutions of Scotland. It was already changing at the earlier date. There was slow but steady economic growth from about 1600 into the 1630s,[1] but from 1638 to 1660 revolution, war and conquest caused great destruction and dislocation. There was the drain of expenditure on war materials, interruption of trade, the permanent loss of young manpower in emigration or death, and war taxation. However, in the long term political and economic stresses speeded up the modernisation of the country, for they reduced the economic strength of the aristocracy and the role of lordship.

The 1660s saw a remarkable recovery, which was sustained for three decades in spite of the setbacks of the Dutch wars. A striking sign of this is the sharp drop in grain prices, approximately of 20 per cent, in the early 1660s, which suggests an easier relationship between food supply and population.[2] The lower prices discouraged landowners from investment in agricultural improvement but drove them to diversify the activities of their estates. The 1670s was a great period for the founding of new burghs and markets, and even though many of these never got off paper, there were some of social and economic significance, which encouraged mobility. In the 1680s the government attempted, with some success, to create new industries sheltered by privileges in regulations and taxation from the chill winds of international competition.[3] There was no general famine in these decades, and transport was able to contain local shortages within manageable proportions. The industrial side of these developments was fragile but set the scene for later growth.

The later seventeenth century saw a series of Acts of Parliament, such as that of 1686 'for winter herding' or that of 1695 'anent Lands lying Runrig'. These could, in the right circumstances, have done much to encourage more effective use of the land.[4] They were passed in the interests of the landowning class in a Parliament dominated by that class but this does not mean that they were in opposition to the interests of those who worked the land. These people, the tenants and subtenants, at least in the Lowlands, appear to have accepted an individualistic ethos even though

2: The Changing Economic and Social Setting

they had to work communally. They were not tied to the land by legal bonds, rights or affection: their relationship with their landowners was by lease or by tenancy 'at will', if they were tenants. Less formal agreements between tenants and subtenants or cottars gave the latter some access to land, and the former some part of their labour input. The system of farm service was for children to leave home early in their teens, if not before, to live and work for other families and to move from one farming household to another.

There is a customary image of a peasant society, with the whole of each household committed to the exploitation of an inherited holding, in some cases in collaboration with other households, and with the land and its main crops regarded not as commercial assets but as an inalienable heritage. If this image had ever been true of lowland Scotland, it had ceased to be so before the seventeenth century. There were still areas where the joint farm, occupied by several tenants with intermixed but individually possessed arable units, dominated the landscape, but this type of settlement had become rare in the most advanced region, the Lothians. More and more tenancies were held by written lease rather than by verbal agreement or by tradition. Labour services were an important part of the rent, and these still bound the tenant and his labour force to make frequent contact with the landowner or his representative, but in both Highlands and Lowlands landowners were trying to enlarge the proportion of the rent due in money. 'Payment in kind' was disappearing and money became the means of settling deals for all classes in the Lowlands. Even relatively humble families were used to handling money, and surprisingly large sums sometimes passed through their hands. This is revealed by occasional large 'voluntary' charitable collections which the Church could extract in times of economic tranquillity (though the Church had a somewhat one-sided understanding of the word 'voluntary') and also by the considerable sums lent by tenants to the economic enterprises of their landowners.[5] The Lowland 'peasantry' was thoroughly monetised, motivated by profit, and held no particular devotion to any individual unit of land.

In the eighteenth century the drive by both landowners and tenants for better land use led to the process of 'enclosure', that is the walling off of individual fields and the separating of holdings. There was also pressure on the cottar class, which over the century was to transform it (at least in the Lowlands) into farm servants or labourers. The existence of cottar holdings had enabled these people and their children to avoid hirings which appeared unattractive, and they were more independent than suited their employers, the tenants. As the single tenancy farm became the norm, it increased the gulf between tenants and cottars or labourers, encouraged more effective use of manpower, and weakened the coherence of rural society. Already in the seventeenth century the gulf between those two farming groups was considerable. The burden of economic insecurity lay almost entirely on the cottars, even though insecurity no longer meant exposure to famine. It was, for instance, very rare for a tenant to become so destitute as to need poor relief. Besides the long established gulf between landowners and tillers of the soil, during the eighteenth century a gulf was opening between tenants and the less privileged group who made up most of the labour force.

These changes enhanced the sense of individualism of those in good economic positions. Landowners ceased to have to maintain personal contact with their tenants or to put pressure on them to fulfil the complex series of obligations laid down in rentals and tacks, and the tenantry when it came to pay its rent entirely in money, was able to exploit the land as best fitted the market economy. Landowners found it profitable to have large farms, and for the same to be true for their tenants. The labourers did not have the link with the land which had given some element of independence to subtenants, nor did they need the labour of their children. The complex economic linkages of early modern society were turning into simple cash transactions in the late eighteenth century.

Population growth after 1750 stimulated food prices and hence agriculture, but since improved agriculture was labour-efficient and could not employ the surplus population, families migrated to urban life and industry. There was thus a rapid increase in mobility, not only of the people themselves, but of markets in goods and in labour skills. Economic and demographic changes were, by 1770, transforming the way of life and the priorities of many in the Lowlands.

Development in the Highlands was slower but similar. Rivalry or hostility between clans, and the confinement of settlement to narrow strips of fertile valley, restricted the movement of people. The level of monetisation was low, though clan chiefs in the later seventeenth century were copying lowland landlords in trying to obtain more of their revenue in cash. We cannot be certain that the desire, so conspicuous in the nineteenth century highland community, for retention of a foothold on land in the area to which people were accustomed was as strongly developed in the previous two centuries:[6] it may have gained in force from cultural isolation, religious extremism and economic collapse. Certainly the readiness of some highlanders to migrate to the cities or overseas, when in the later eighteenth century they were free to do so, suggests that by then economic prosperity mattered more to such people than retention of a plot of land.

It is not clear whether the highlanders of the later seventeenth century shared the same economic motivation as the lowland community, partly because their individual motivation is obscured to us by their obligations to their clan chief. This tie was destroyed in the attack on clanship after the 1745 Jacobite rising, and by the later eighteenth century neither highlander nor lowlander considered his relationship to his landlord, for that is what chiefs had become, as involving personal loyalty. The more independent-minded may well have felt exasperated at still having to fulfil services to landowners as part of the tenurial bargain.[7] But lordship continued, even in the Lowlands into the early eighteenth century, to have aspects of authority and obligation not solely based on tenurial relationships, and in the Highlands chiefly dominance, even if resented, remained a conspicuous feature until the changes forced by the events of 1745.

The main change of the early eighteenth century was the 1707 treaty of union with England. The Scottish motivation for this was the weakness of the economy, as demonstrated by the hardships of the 1690s. The treaty left the Scottish Church and the Scottish legal system apparently untouched. In reality, however, the Church was not immune to interference: one of the early actions of the new Parliament of Great Britain was to establish some level of religious toleration for protestant dissent in Scotland, and to accompany this by the reintroduction of lay patronage over church appointments. The legal system was affected more gradually by the introduction of a system of appeals to the House of Lords as supreme court. Scots law at the time of union needed new features which would recognise the enhanced political significance of the gentry in opposition to the powers of the aristocracy, and it

2: The Changing Economic and Social Setting

received them in judicial decisions over a wide front.[8] Economic development fostered the growth of mercantile law. Union hastened these developments.

The trend towards individualism was apparent in other areas of life. Modernisation of the criminal law was one of these. As in other parts of Europe, law in Scotland had combined popular practices and traditions with the more modern concept of specific orders emanating from the central government. Offences might well be absorbed by the local community without penalty, since overt action could lead to revenge by the offender or by his kin. In the Crown's courts different principles controlled the procedures and penalties for people of wealth and status from those applicable to the common people, for the payment of compensation by offenders or their kin was a swifter and more sure way to end a feud than was any State-imposed penalty. Increasing professionalism among lawyers and judges and the influence of the Church drove the change towards the concept of crime as a breach of an explicit rule, and that penalties should be the same for all. The idea of crime as an offence, the offensiveness of which did not lie in the wickedness of the intent behind it, was encouraged by the Church. Criminal acts were a direct offence to God and, unpunished, a menace to society. Law thus became more uniform and penalties harsher in the seventeenth century. At the same time a more professional lawyers' code of what was and what was not admissible evidence provided some protection for the accused.

The trend towards individualism necessarily weakened lordship. In any case the power of the aristocracy never recovered after the period of revolution. In 1647 the Church had showed that it could prevent the tenantry supporting its lords. In the Restoration period there were occasions when landowners claimed that they could not control their tenants in matters such as church attendance and other issues of conscience. By the late seventeenth century even a highland chief could not assume that his clansmen would automatically follow him with arms in every alliance he might make. In the Jacobite risings of the eighteenth century men followed their chiefs, but often only after threats, and many deserted whenever opportunity showed.

An important legal change of the seventeenth century was the idea of criminal responsibility of women. Before then, responsibility for offences committed by women had lain with their governing menfolk, with the father of an unmarried woman, the husband of a wife, and with the son if she was a widow. This indicates group rather than individual responsibility, and suggests that women were seen as chattels. In a system where a widespread kin could be called upon to make compensation for crime, it was of no particular interest that the criminal was a woman. Both Reformation and Counter Reformation had emphasised personal responsibility by both sexes, but the criminal law was slow to reflect this. The striking exception was witchcraft, where some 80 per cent of those accused were women. Over a thousand were executed in the seventeenth century, and since accusations were likely to flare in any place which had already experienced the witchcraft craze, there were lowland areas where any sharp-tongued woman who did not have influential relations was at real risk.[9]

At the same time both the criminal and the civil law had difficulty in accepting women as witnesses. A surprising amount of the time of educated legal manpower in court was spent in arguing this issue.[10] A common compromise was that women could bear witness only on events for which it was unlikely that there would be male witnesses,[11] although they were accepted as witnesses in all Commissary Court cases and in church courts. When concealed pregnancy led to a dead infant, infanticide was always assumed, and women were questioned as witnesses in the criminal courts.

Dogma made it clear that women had souls of equal concern to God as those of men, but they were still second-class citizens in the eyes of both Church and State. The revulsion shown in the 1560 Confession of Faith over the Roman Catholic practice of allowing women to baptise extended further than the conveying of the sacrament, for baptism was available only to infants whom a male sponsor would present. If a woman was in trouble with her kirk session her husband might be included in the reproof, presumably on the grounds that he had not adequately controlled her. A husband was expected to rule his household, by violence if need be. The Church acquiesced in the idea of male superiority, but made attempts to modify the violence. A minister would reprove a man for exceeding the accepted level of marital violence if it was inflicted in public, or if the woman made it public by screaming or running away, and severe violence would bring such behaviour under the head of scandal. In June 1695, in Dumbarton, Duncan Campbell had added to his offences of slander and drunkenness on the sabbath, hitting his wife when out of doors with such force that she thought her hearing had been damaged, and he was ordered by the presbytery to do penance. In Cameron, November 1697, Andrew Robertson was summoned to the session for striking his wife and setting his foot upon her. He stated that he only 'drew a foot out under her because she arose not soon enough at his bidding' and added, 'will you deny me that obedience due to me by my wife?'. He was recommended to bear with his wife with meekness and exhorted to behave more circumspectly. A man would also be reproved if chastisement took place on Sunday. Usually any reproof of a husband would be accompanied by a reproof of the wife for having provoked him. If a man retorted angrily to inquiry by a kirk session into his behaviour, or refused to carry out its orders, the session would maintain its pressure but without further reproof; whereas if a woman did the same she would receive a strongly worded reproof.

In Caithness women guilty of sexual offences in the seventeenth century and early years of the eighteenth were often beaten, but not the men. In burghs in the eighteenth century prostitutes might be flogged and forced to leave town, but no action would be taken against their customers. A woman offender might be labelled a whore or common strumpets but there was no derogatory word for a man whose offences repeatedly brought him before the session.

Yet women were not surplus to the economy. They were a vital part of the work force for their skill, suppleness and (within limits) their strength. They did the outdoor jobs that involved stooping, or were wet or messy. They did not usually form part of the group ploughing, nor act as herds, but they worked in the sowing and harrowing. In harvest they were the reapers, using sickles.[12] They did the pulling of flax, the carrying of peats, the whole range of dairy work, the spinning, cooking and such minimal cleaning and washing as was expected, and collaborated with men in winnowing, malting and brewing, and retting the flax. In mining they went underground along with the men to carry up the coal, and in other industries they did much of the unskilled but tiring work.

Poverty and lack of possessions forced the sexes into close contact. Most houses were of one room, measuring not more than 20 by 14 feet,[13] and at least until well into the eighteenth century these were undivided rooms. Only then was Scotland affected by the 'domestic revolution' diagnosed by Dr Hoskins in England, in which a sudden change of life style occurred, with the purchase of good furniture, the improvement of house structure, the achievement of some minimal level of privacy by the creation of extra rooms, and the making of window curtains.[14] The few household inventories which survive from tenants and cottars show that in the early eighteenth century even reasonably prosperous farmers would have almost no place of comfort except their beds, and almost no change of linen.[15] Box beds, common in the nineteenth century, which made a division in the room, only appeared in the mid-eighteenth century. So did luxury purchases such as oak tables, chests of drawers and mirrors. For most of the period of our study these features did not obtain, and the people lived in a world where privacy and cleanliness were impossible.

By contrast the better off lairds from the late seventeenth century onwards enjoyed luxurious accommodation, fine furniture and elegant houses and gardens. The gentry gave up living in tower houses, for the most part in the Restoration period, since law and order made for less need of verticality and more ease. The Scottish upper classes had been slow, by European standards, to abandon their medieval military functions. In the seventeenth century most of the aristocracy had at least a dilettante command of troops, though some had only a vague idea of how to handle weapons, let alone how to deploy soldiers in battle. By the 1680s the situation had changed in the Lowlands. Military activity had become a specific career, in which only a few were engaged. The sword might still be worn, but simply as a sign of gentility, an indicator that the wearer was entitled to settle disputes by its use.

Promotion of the lairds had been the aim of James VI who had not managed to achieve it, though he had created the office of Justice of the Peace, which was to become one of the instruments by which these men controlled society. Charles I had had a similar aim, and his settlement of teind reinforced the lairds' position. In the mid-seventeenth they moved into the power vacuum created when the aristocracy were defeated and disciplined by the church party. The upper range of the lairds, those who were tenants in chief of the Crown, supported the independence of Parliament from 1688, even though the political groups within which they worked were controlled by the great magnates. Union with England completed the rise of the lairds by turning the ambitions of the aristocracy to London. Political and military careers had to be pursued there, and even some legal ones. It was in London that whatever spoils the government had to distribute were to be sought. The aristocrats capable of an important role moved from Scotland and left effective power there to the lairds.

The word 'laird' covers a wide range of landowning income. At the top were men of estates equivalent in size and wealth to those of the lesser aristocracy, with some interchange between their ranks. Examples of such elevation were the Murrays of Scone, ennobled in 1757, and the Elliots of Minto, who had benefited by marriage with an heiress and reached the House of Lords in 1797. In some cases a laird in this group might become the only landowner in a parish, with a very powerful voice in its affairs. Then there were the owners of moderate estates, which would provide, unimproved, an income of between £100 and £1,000 a year. Finally there were the men to whom Sir Walter Scott gave the label of 'bonnet laird', and who were more officially referred to as 'proprietors of single farms', a group of economic standing no higher than some of the greater tenants. These men were under economic pressure, and becoming fewer in the later eighteenth century, but were still of considerable social significance. Often they had a taste for a larger income than a single farm could provide, and would rent out their land and move into the professions, usually law. The advocates and judges of late seventeenth and eighteenth century Scotland were almost entirely drawn from the ranks of the medium and small landowners.

In spite of differences in wealth the class of landowners had status and unity, reinforced by intermarriage. A common feature throughout the class was the aspiration for gracious living. According to Sir John Sinclair, there were, at the end of the eighteenth century, almost 400 large estates worth over £2,500 a year, just over a thousand middling ones and over 6,000 giving less than £600 a year. Dr Timperley, who is probably a more accurate source, confirms these figures as nearly true for 1770: her numbers are 336 large estates, 1,100 middling and over 6,100 small.[16] These figures cannot be directly translated into landed families, for such families might hold land in different counties, but they give some idea of the numbers in the class.

The different types of estate were unevenly distributed. Large estates dominated the scene in the Borders and in East Lothian. 'Bonnet lairds', even though they did not control much of the total acreage, were numerous in Lanarkshire, Galloway and Ayrshire, Banffshire, Bute and the central Lowlands, and fairly common in Fife and Caithness.[17]

Landowners often had the right to appoint the minister and had considerable influence over the appointment of a schoolmaster. They were liable to pay stipend and schoolmaster's salary, as well as the costs of repair of church and manse. By being uncooperative over appointments or slow in payment, they could make life very uncomfortable for a parish which displeased them.

Some members of the landed class were involved in the expanding commerce of the eighteenth century, or in banking. When rents had been paid in kind, rather than in money, the need to sell agricultural surpluses caused landowners to develop mercantile skills and a network of contacts. Unlike English values, this did not detract from their social prestige: Scottish respectability did not depend on the absence of a link with trade, but the reality of a link, however slight, with landowning. Younger sons might also go into trade as an alternative to the army or to government service, and the professional posts which expanded rapidly in the eighteenth century, in medicine, the navy, and the universities, were frequently held by men linked to land. The Church ministry might receive some recruitment from the landed classes, but for the most part was self-sustaining, a hereditary caste.[18] Merchant houses and craftsmen's workshops also kept as much family continuity as the risks of bankruptcy allowed. These semi-closed groups made for a society in which people knew their place well, and held to it without any discomfort in the consciousness of the social superiority and the reality of power in the landowning class.

The eighteenth century could be called the century of the lairds, for the landed gentry dominated the law, the economy, culture and society. These men did not rest idle in their position. They inherited (literally) a country backward in economy, dominated by territorial magnates and bullied by a dogmatic and intransigent clergy. They transformed it into an active participant in social change and economic growth, contributing significantly to the industrial revolution and to the eighteenth century intellectual movement which we call the Enlightenment.[19]

The landed class came, somewhat grudgingly, to co-operate with the Church in

2: The Changing Economic and Social Setting

making the poor law of Scotland into a working system, at least in the Lowlands. Much of what was in the statute book on the support of the needy and the disciplining of vagrants was never put into practice, and so ceased, through the Scottish legal principle of 'desuetude', to have any authority. But in the period of Whig dominance in the mid-seventeenth century the Church had secured an Act of Parliament handing the management of relief to its courts,[20] and this Act marks the start of all practices which could be called a poor law. The aristocracy was then politically in eclipse, and in some lowland parishes the ministers were able insist on assessment and levies (i.e. ratepaying) from landowners, for a time at least. From then on lowland parishes regularly worked some system of support for the infirm and indigent, and received legacies to sustain this work, plus the fines for misbehaviour. The funds of a parish were normally known as the poor's money, even though they were used also to support the parish officer and clerk, the clerks of the higher courts, and to provide for necessities such as communion equipment, and minor conveniences such as a church porch. In the famine of the 1690s pressure from the Privy Council through the system of county government supported ministers in gaining help from landowners, and many parishes were able to impose assessment on landowners. They were aided in this by an Act of Parliament which shared the landowners' burden with the tenantry.[21] This was one of the few enactments on poor relief which took effect. On the whole the system developed under the authority of the Church, rather than of the State.

In the eighteenth century the relief system in the Lowlands was capable of supporting the obvious cases of need, but at a low level. There were campaigns by county governing groups to make it adequate, and also to force parishes to control vagrancy. In the south and south-east of Scotland this led to most parishes being assessed (i.e. rated) on a permanent basis by the end of the century, but assessment was rare and occasional in the north and north-east. However, in these areas the needs of those severely destitute were often partly met by special collections. In periods of crop failure, notably the very bad harvests of 1740 and 1782, landowners in both north and south made generous gifts and collected subscriptions to subsidise grain purchases and keep the population from starvation. In 1782 the Highlands were bailed out by grain left over from the War of the American Revolution, but in normal times the weakness of parish structure there, and the tenuous government control meant that poor relief barely existed. Parishes might make an occasional dole of a few shillings, but were not able to support those with no resources.

Thus, lowland Scotland developed a system of effective relief in the eighteenth century, but one with limitations. Landowners liked to think of it as a matter of generous giving rather than legal obligation, and in the north came to view assessment with hostility.[22] There was a struggle for control of parish funds in the mid-eighteenth century between landowners and the Church, but in practice the legal victory of the landowners made little difference. Since relief funds were never lavish, there were no major policy decisions for landowners to influence, and they were not interested in the detailed work of distribution. The allowances given in a parish would keep an elderly and infirm person from starvation, care for orphans and foundlings until they were ready for service or apprenticeship (and even provide medical aid for them after they had entered service), sustain the insane in some comfort, give partial help to men whose losses put their earning power at risk and bury pensioners with seemly rites. But the poor law never established a right to relief in a claimant. Occasionally lawyers might bring a case for a claimant in the sheriff court, and the decision might order a specified level of parish support, but the general principle was that the kirk session accepted an obligation to support the poor of which it was the judge.[23] This absence of paupers' rights, while it meant that Scotland did not have to develop the structure of settlement law which attempted to control labour movement in England, also meant that there was no obligation on a Scottish parish to support illegitimate children. A parish might well give an allowance to a nursing mother of a legitimate or illegitimate child who had no other resource while her nursing prevented her from employment, but this was merely a temporary aid. This absence of support for bastards, other than foundlings, meant that the moral control which the Church exercised over sexual affairs had little mercenary motivation: it was based simply on Calvinist dogma.

Already in the seventeenth century both lairds and nobility sought to increase the yield of their estates. They were involved together in the drive for more market outlets in the 1670s, supported the attempts of Privy Council and Parliament to expand the range of industries in the 1680s, and encouraged linen manufacture on their estates and the marketing of cattle in England. Linen was to become the dominant industry in Scotland. It often provided the money with which tenants paid their rent, increased the resources of many poor households by giving profitable work to women and children and, since it was an industry aimed at export, had a marked influence on the improvement of roads and the expansion of market activity. Between the 1720s and the 1770s the value of linen reaching the open market, and much was done to private contract, went up over five times. Much of the effect of this change can only be guessed at, for the firms who organised its transport or sale were often too small to leave records. But it clearly caused a major change in the availability of markets, although not until the eighteenth century.

Many of the new burghs created in and after the 1670s never had anything which could be called urban life, and new industries did not take root. The idea, expressed in an Act of 1672, that vagrants could be made into an effective labour force for new industries was, understandably, nothing but a mirage. What is of importance in the various plans and schemes is the idea, not only of profit, but of economic development as desirable in itself. New ideas had more effect in agriculture, and several Acts of the newly independent parliament at the end of the century gave landowners a freer hand in the management of their estates. As we saw earlier, though landowners were not ready yet to undertake the drastic reorganisation which would really send up output, yet they were prepared to weaken traditional relationships in the search for economic gain.[24]

It was thus only in the eighteenth century that the agricultural revolution came about in Scotland, and it was well into that century before money rents replaced rents in kind and in services. Rents in kind dictated the cultivation pattern that could be used by tenants, and so fostered their dependency. Services such as labour in harvest, or 'carriages', which meant the labour and carts to carry the landowner's goods, were a similar shackle upon the tenant's ideas of self-betterment.

Landowners simply could not see that a freer use of the tenants' time could enhance their productivity. One of the first members of landed society to put forward a written argument for 'improvement' (changes in the method of production) was William Mackintosh of Borlum. His *An Essay on Ways and Means for Inclosing, Fallowing, Planting etc....*, of 1729, claimed that the introduction of fences and the

2: The Changing Economic and Social Setting

separation of farms would be an expenditure which would lead rapidly to profit. He also went on to argue against 'services' but had to admit that he could not see how landowners would ever manage without having their peats cut and brought in by their tenants. Where the most adventurous thinker could not see that paid labour would become available to fill this gap, agricultural reorganisation was bound to be delayed. Borlum was, in fact, in advance of most of landed society in perceiving that some of the economic rights which seemed advantageous to landowners, particularly the right to labour services, might be holding back productivity from which landowners might gain more markedly. Another early 'improver', John Cockburn of Ormiston, shows his limited appreciation of this point, for though he did much to promote the security of his more successful tenants, he still insisted on using his right to have and use a dovecote, in other words to provide himself with meat at the expense of his tenants' corn.

The most striking area of development in the first half of the eighteenth century was in the economic infrastructure, that is in transport, communications and financial services. This ground work was responsible for the remarkable growth of the third quarter. A rough indication of this growth can be seen in the 40 per cent increase in Scotland's home manufactured exports,[25] but more significant in social terms was the corresponding growth in internal trade, which cannot be easily measured. Much of the growth was based on small scale cottage production, which transformed domestic life for many households. The change in the quality of transport facilities, and the use made of them, also had great impact on the lives of the people. Towns, which expanded faster in eighteenth-century Scotland than anywhere else in Europe, grew in scale and changed markedly in the services which they offered. People moved from place to place, sometimes of necessity but also often of choice, and their movements could no longer be controlled by the system of 'testificats', certificates of good behaviour given by the kirk session of the parish from which someone was moving, and without which the parish of his proposed stay would not receive him. In the second half of the century kirk sessions cease to refer to these documents except to verify marriages. An important element in the control of the people had been lost.

This increased mobility of the mass of the people also lessened the influence of the landowning class, even if it did not affect its legal rights. An evicted farm tenant could find openings elsewhere: the towns needed more and more labour. The transport system itself, the roads and bridges, the carting system, the inns and stage coaches, all needed hands. Later came wider prospects for the dissatisfied and adventurous in the expansion of the American colonies. Scotland provided much of the surge of emigration to America in the 1770s, sending whole farming families into the unknown. One of the motives which inspired this movement was the desire to be free of the burdens of rent and services and gain control of the management of a piece of land. A marked streak of individualism sustained this movement.

Individualism produced a different response in the upper class. The intellectual fashion of the day was to become known as the Enlightenment: its basic theory was a development from the work of writers of the seventeenth century which has become known as civic humanism. This theory laid down secular principles of moral action for the citizen. It defined the citizen as an independent man, i.e. a landowner, excluding those who relied on others for employment or tenure: 'to qualify for... citizenship the individual must be master of his own household, proprietor along with his own equals of the only arms permitted to be borne in wars... and possessor of property.'[26] Citizenship was exclusively the possession of adult male landowner heads of households. Civic humanism confirmed the widely held belief that the function of the State was to protect landed property, a belief actively used by the landed class at this time since it alone had representation in Parliament and it also supplied the judiciary. Using the theory of civic humanism men were able to discuss morals without reference to Calvinist dogma. It was not so much that dogma was denied or refuted: most of the discussants of humanist issues would have assented to Calvinism. But the whole body of argument was bypassed in much the same way as it was in the world of the late nineteenth and early twentieth century universities. Christian morality subsumed many of the historical and political judgements of academics then, but was not necessarily expressed.

Landed society did not make the Enlightenment on its own. There was a powerful current entering it from the professions, particularly the professoriate and the clergy. Early in the century a transformation of the universities of Scotland began with the creation of the Edinburgh medical school and the placing of Alexander Monro as the first professor of anatomy. Monro has left us a book-sized document of advice, in the form of a letter to his daughter, which, though it discusses many aspects of behaviour, makes no explicit reference to revealed religion.[27] For working purposes the professional theorising of the great men in the medical schools was conceived entirely in terms of natural philosophy, not of dogma. The 1740s saw the emergence of a powerful though small group of young clergy concerned to promote freedom in artistic and intellectual culture, who were to be known as the leaders of the Moderate party in the Church.[28]

David Hume was the protagonist of those sceptical, or even hostile, to theology and organised religion. The other conspicuous figures of the Enlightenment did not oppose Calvinism, but most of them avoided expatiating on it. It was feasible for Adam Smith in his analysis of the economy to speak of an 'invisible hand' without regarding it as part of an anthropomorphic God. The achievement of the Enlightenment was to develop the natural and social sciences in their own terms, as subject to their own discoverable laws.

These intellectual and economic changes did not come about painlessly, or with harmony of opinion. The Moderate clerics downplayed the idea of predestination and were attacked for this by John Witherspoon and other dogmatic Calvinists, but they did not see how sermons on those lines would help their flocks to lead more Christian lives.[29]

Even as early as the late seventeenth century some elements of landed society resented the political and moral claims of the clergy. For instance, the professional lawyers, almost all landowning, were unwilling to aid in prosecutions for witchcraft and other ecclesiastical cases. In 1696 the Court of Justiciary had sentenced a young man of undistinguished birth, one Thomas Aikenhead, to death for blasphemy, but might have considered a reprieve if so urged by the Edinburgh clergy. These ministers, so far from seeking mercy, urged immediate execution to prevent any intervention from the Crown in London.[30] In 1704 a group of Pittenweem women was accused of witchcraft, but it was alleged that a local minister had obtained a confession by beating one of them.[31] At this interval of time it is not possible to sort out the full details of this sordid and violent case, which ended with a lynching, but these accusations of 'barbarous severitys' by ministers show strong upper class hostility to the clergy. Anticlericalism, in the seventeenth century usually directed

2: The Changing Economic and Social Setting

only at clerical influence on political matters, became more open and widespread because of the intolerant behaviour of the remnant of 'outed' ministers which had gained control of the General Assembly and was purging the Church of all who had accepted episcopacy. The Act of Union and the 1712 Toleration Act, opposed by the clergy because the statutes would, and did, reduce clerical power, made possible greater openness of resistance to clerical demands. But it is striking that the lawyers, though they were able to frustrate most witchcraft prosecutions, never denounced the legal basis of the offence until it had been abolished by statute in 1736.

There were new as well as old grounds for friction between landowners and clergy. Presbyteries were taking as a standard for manses, which the landowners would have to pay for, a much larger and more solidly built house than in the past. There were often parish issues over grazing for the minister's horse. In 1749 various presbyteries and synods put before the General Assembly their view that the incomes of many ministers were inadequate. It was claimed that the cost of living had risen since stipends had been fixed in the first half of the seventeenth century. It would be more accurate to say that, since stipends had been fixed in grain, and grain prices had fallen in the 1660s, the clergy's purchasing power had declined. The century or so which had elapsed had seen the production of more types of goods, and a rise in the wages of labourers and servants. There was now an established middle class life style to which the clergy aspired. But stipends were levied off rents, and landowners in many counties loudly opposed the Augmentation scheme. When the General Assembly ignored these hostilities and went ahead with the scheme the landed members of Parliament secured its consignation to the category of indefinite postponement in 1751, but not before a good deal of intemperate language on both sides had been aired in the Assembly and the press.[32]

This was not the only mid-century clash between lay and clerical. A series of law suits over the handling of the parish funds for poor relief, which appear to have had a linked organisation, led to judicial decisions in 1751 which dismayed the ministers and surprised even some judges. They asserted that the landowners of a parish had by natural right complete control over all its funds, and they also laid down impractical restrictions on what could be done with parish money. However, in the long run little was changed, because it was in no-one's interests to wreck the existing system of support for the poor.[33]

If the laity were anti-clerical, then how did the clergy feel towards the laity? In the 1750s and 1760s many ministers were furious at the powers and behaviour of landowners. It was a new experience for the Scottish Church to discover that lay society might not, even outwardly, conform to its views. Sermons and pamphlets from this period bewail a serious fall off in moral standards and in church attendance on the part of the gentry,[34] but such writings give more evidence of ecclesiastical pique than of deterioration in lay behaviour. The protection of the known sceptic, David Hume, from ecclesiastical censure or worse is usually one of the grievances, but the frustration of the Augmentation scheme ranks was a deeper resentment. For instance, Patrick Bannerman's sermon preached to the synod at Stirling in 1751 states that 'Infidelity, Scepticism, or an absolute Indifference about all Religion, prevail so much among Persons of Rank and Fashion, that these have become the Characteristics by which Men would distinguish themselves from the Vulgar', and James Oswald, preaching at the opening of the General Assembly in 1766, specifically attacked men of high rank, and accused them of 'contemptuous neglect of religious duties'. Nevertheless, William Creech in his 'Letters to Sir John Sinclair' specifically stated that 'In 1763 – It was fashionable to go to church. Sunday was strictly observed by all ranks.'[35]

The literature brings out the gulf between clerics and landed society, and also reveals divisions within the Church. The political Revolution of 1688–89 had marginalised the episcopal faction, but since these included most of the ministry of Aberdeenshire and the north-east, there was considerable confusion and disorder in that region. The Episcopalian Church, which these dissenters formed, did not dissent from the Calvinism of the establishment but its political links with Jacobitism put it under difficulties, and after the 1715 rebellion some proscription. There was also an extremist covenanting sect, mainly in the south-west. But still, for the first third of the eighteenth century, the established Presbyterian Church was very nearly national in its scope, and hard line Calvinism prevailed.

There were, however, some doctrinal differences, mainly associated with an English book of seventeenth-century origin, *The Marrow of Modern Divinity*, republished in 1718. This book emphasised free grace, thus denying supralapsarianism. Grace could be made available to any sinner who sincerely sought it, and was not limited to a predetermined minority. The book was condemned by the General Assembly in 1720, but there was always a party from then on uneasy over the official expression of the Church's theology, the Westminster Confession.

The Marrow controversy was one of the strands which led to the first open secession of a presbyterian group from the Church in the 1730s, but this group's protest was not over free grace: it was on the relative ways in which suppression of The Marrow and of other forms of deviant opinion had been treated, and, behind that, the readiness of the Assembly to accept lay patronage in appointments imposed by the State.[36]

Patronage had been reintroduced, after its abolition in 1690, by the British Parliament in an Act which was not only offensive to the Church but also a violation of the accepted terms of the Union of 1707. This had included a Scottish statute affirming the independence of the Church. Patronage issues could create great local heat, rituals of protest and sometimes serious resistance to imposed ministers and continuing rifts within congregations. They enhanced the hostility between the landed class, which supported patronage, and the 'popular' party in the Church. The existence of even the small, but tightly organised and excessively self-righteous 'Original Secession', an alternative presbyterian church, was bound to weaken the authority of the Established Church. The Original Secession was distinctly 'holier than thou', so that though it denounced 'sapless and lifeless descanting upon the moral virtues', there was no likelihood of it becoming a refuge for those who could not take the discipline of the Establishment. It had no appeal to moral deviants.

It was the second secession, that of the 1750s, again taking its start on the topic of patronage and the insistence of the Assembly in overriding presbyteries, which created a communion, the Relief Church, in 1761, open to those unhappy with hard line Calvinism. No doctrinal requirements were placed on attendance at this Church's communion. Even before this the issue of free grace had been raised through a series of revival meetings. The first of these was held in the open at Cambuslang in 1742. The revivals became associated with the visit of George Whitefield, a leading preacher of the eighteenth-century evangelical movement. They brought converts to accept a serious commitment to religion; in so doing they

2: The Changing Economic and Social Setting

accentuated the gulf between the upper class and popular religion. It was not coincidence that Cambuslang was a parish with persistent bad relations between the heritors (mainly episcopalian) and the kirk session, relations which were revealed when it became one of the parishes picked on for a court case over the relative rights of the two groups. Landowners regarded the prospect of a religious revival on their land – and the 'Great Wark' of Cambuslang was repeated annually – much as a modern landowner would regard a pop festival on his. There would be thousands of people gathered together, noise, emotional scenes, damage to fences, excrement, petty theft, and the general distraction of the workforce from its duties.[37]

The various secessions and revivals were evidence of genuine popular religious enthusiasm. We do not know the numbers affected, but they were considerable. It has been alleged that as many as 100,000 adhered to the Relief Church in 1765, but this is only a guess.[38] In any case, it is the existence of the communion, rather than its size, which mattered, because it ended the exclusive acceptance of the Westminster Confession.

The mid-eighteenth century thus saw the development in different sections of society of two drastically opposed currents of thought. On one hand, fanned by the revival meetings, a theology more inviting and individualist than traditional Calvinism was offering participation and support to the unpropertied part of society. On the other hand, educated men could enter into the new exploration of the physical world and of the social influences of mankind which was the Enlightenment.

The Enlightenment was particularly the expression of ideas among the landed gentry and professional men of Edinburgh and Glasgow. Its main foci were the clubs in the cities; clubs for the discussion of specific intellectual matters and clubs concerned to promote the economy of Scotland. (Two of these still survive: the Royal Society of Edinburgh and the Highland Society.) A striking illustration of the range of interest expressed in these clubs, and the intellectual distance covered since the seventeenth century, is shown in an essay 'On Venery', written by the minister Robert Wallace. In this paper, for which no contemporary references survive, Wallace urged that it be recognised that the sexual urge was as strong in women as in men, and that there was an inevitable sexual element in all close relationships between people of different sex. He suggested that a system of trial marriage be set up for young people to avoid marital disharmony. He felt that fornication should be discouraged but not regarded as a stigma. The most interesting aspect of this paper is that one of the more influential members of the clergy should feel free to discuss sexual matters without having to denounce deviancy.[39]

The club life was available to those ministers who could maintain contact with the dominant cities. A small group of such men in and around Edinburgh formed the core of the Moderate party in the Church, sharing in the culture of the Enlightenment and promoting the policy of co-operation between Church and civil society. Their existence polarised issues within the Church, and the Popular and Moderate parties took opposing sides on almost every significant issue. The Moderates were numerically in a minority, but for several decades following their emergence in 1752 they managed to dominate the decisions of the General Assembly by the votes of the gentry members.[40]

Given the frequent occasions of hostility between 'Popular' ecclesiastics and landowners, this fact enhanced the bitterness between the parties. John Witherspoon, later to make his mark as first Principal of Princeton University, and less successfully as a land speculator in the new settlements in America, anonymously labelled his opponents as 'professed unbelievers, desiring to retain the name of Christian'. Such invective would lead later historians to believe that the Moderates had abandoned Calvinism, and with it church discipline, but the evidence of kirk session registers disproves this. For instance, Alexander Carlyle of Inveresk, a leading Moderate, can be seen in his parish's records to have been a conscientious minister particularly concerned with the welfare of the poor. His comments on his parish in the OSA also show a strong sympathy with the secular culture and aspirations of ordinary people.[41]

Carlyle's concerns, and the friendship network of the Moderates, reveal the real change occurring in people's minds, the acceptance of secular interests as permitted manifestations of individualism. Among the participants in the Enlightenment were men who accepted traditional Calvinism, but who were prepared to be friends with the acknowledged sceptic, David Hume, and Hume had made a very powerful attack on the claims of the Church to divine authority.

Humanitarianism was another current of influential thought, not necessarily associated with the main figures of the Enlightenment, particularly among some of the lawyers. These men had modified the severity of the criminal law on certain topics, most notably, as will be shown in Chapter 3, on the definitions of incest. There are other signs of humanitarian ethic, for instance the letters written to the *Scots Magazine* in 1757, arguing that it was fear of church discipline which led girls to infanticide, and urging that the procedures be made less intimidating.[42] In 1785, in a collection of criminal cases of the last two centuries, the distinguished lawyer, Hugh Arnot, attacked the presumption of guilt of infanticide which held in cases of concealment of pregnancy. That other lawyers were uneasy on this matter is shown by the drastic statutory modification of the law which took place in the early nineteenth century. In 1770, however, an Act of the General Assembly denouncing clandestine marriage stressed the dangerous social and moral effects which could follow carelessness or leniency in the examination by kirk sessions of claims to be married.[43] This Act shows that many in the Church wished to see discipline more systematically observed, and is a reminder that humanitarianism could be used to support severity as well as to oppose it.

The Church's capacity to repress had clearly become reduced in all classes of society. Signs of an overt and non-intellectual interest in sexuality, expressed in ways which at the beginning of the century the Church would certainly have denounced, can be seen. Surviving chapbooks, roughly dateable to this period, without being openly lewd show an independence of the views of the Church on fornication. In one of the most famous, *Jockey and Maggie's Courtship*,[44] the mother of the young man in trouble expresses a view that was to be very common in the high illegitimacy area of the north-east in the mid-nineteenth century: the man was praised as 'neither a thief nor a horse-dealer', and cheered by the reflection that 'ye're no the first that has done it, and ye'll no be the last'. His own statement was simply an unwillingness to do penance in public. The songs of Robert Burns reflect a rich tradition of bawdy, and since singing is a social affair, show that there were places and times where the expression of undisguised sexuality was acceptable.

Sexuality, not merely overt but ostentatious, in the upper class is revealed by the surviving documents of an erotic and voyeuristic club in Anstruther, Fife, confined, by the level of subscription required, to men of substance: lairds, merchants and the local officials of the customs service. This body held regular meetings from the

2: The Changing Economic and Social Setting

1720s until well on in the nineteenth century. Papers relating to it occur in four separate sets of aristocratic estate archives now lodged in the Scottish Record Office.[45] It is difficult to believe that a society with such a high social profile in its membership, meeting regularly in a very small town with some score of local worthies attending, and with local girls hired for the occasion, could have been kept secret. But we have not found any denunciation of the organisation in the records of either parish or presbytery.

Enlightenment thinkers had expressed an appreciation of the variety of human aspirations. Without necessarily sharing the philosophy that sustained this view, many sections of society by the later eighteenth century were prepared to accept that there were areas of life in which human participation was normal, even when these were in conflict with the views of organised religion. The expression of the Shorter Catechism, that the whole duty of man was to glorify God and enjoy Him for ever, simply did not fit their mental systems.

All these developments were to overturn Church discipline in the 1770s–80s, and first and foremost was the new ethos of humanitarianism and individualism, an ethos that was also gaining ground in England and elsewhere.[46] It was well shown in a letter published in 1780 in the *Scots Magazine*. The writer objected to a parish attempting to exercise discipline by advertising in the press about a missing woman, thought to be pregnant. The letter denounced this as a 'flagrant violation of decency' which would never have been inflicted on a girl of higher social status.[47]

Relaxation of discipline was not universal, however. Some parish ministers continued to enforce, or attempt to enforce, the old severe discipline into the 1780s and beyond. An often quoted example of this, because it involved Robert Burns, was the incumbency of the Reverend William Auld, minister of Mauchline, Ayrshire, from 1742 to 1791. But, as is also well known, the attempt of his kirk session to penalise the minor landowner Gavin Hamilton for not attending church, breaches of Sabbath behaviour and failure to hold family prayers, failed in the presbytery.[48]

Calvinism itself was altered by the new tide of evangelicalism. Calvinism in Scotland had stressed the importance of the community, and (as explained in Chapter 1) enforced discipline as part of the community's claim to be godly and saved. By contrast, the evangelism of the early nineteenth century stressed the conversion, inspiration and commitment of the individual Christian and that individual's personal relationship with God. Morality was still important, but there was no particular merit in public penance; it did not ensure the salvation of the congregation and might even encourage spiritual pride on the part of observers. Perhaps it was under this influence that early in the nineteenth century the Church of Scotland started to discourage the practice of public discipline.[49]

The increasing mobility of the population was striking. Movement could involve minor journeying to markets, which now were much more frequent and busier, marriage at a greater distance than in the past, temporary or long-term movement for work or emigration overseas. It was most conspicuous culturally when Highlanders came to live and work in the Lowlands, but this was just one facet. The change is perhaps best, though fictionally, described in John Galt's novel, *Annals of the Parish*. Urban expansion, new centres of industry, the erection and successful management of turnpikes, all bear witness to the flow of people to new places and new opportunities and to a new scale of urban concentration.[50] There was bound to come a time when the Church's detective work, based on personal knowledge and by

Girls in Trouble

correspondence with distant ministers, simply could not maintain the level of information required for effective discipline. Let one minister in a big town give up the attempt to keep track of incomers, and intelligence was lost to the entire clerical network.

By 1770 The Church of Scotland had been abandoned by perhaps 100,000 people, those adhering to dissenting presbyterian communions. This did not directly damage discipline since many of these dissenting communities had even higher standards of morality than the Church of Scotland, and in any case that Church still considered itself entitled and obliged to exercise discipline over those not of its communion. But it made a further dent in the capacity of the Church to trace individuals, since the normal bonds of communication were weakened.

The weakening of discipline was usually first shown in the readiness of a session to accept extra money, above the level of fine, often specifically labelled for the poor, instead of public appearances. This was not a totally new feature: in 1585 the Provost of Elgin, while confessing his fornication to the session, had argued that 'repentance consistit not in the external gestoir of the bodie. but in the hart', and had been let off external gestures in return for repairing the north window of the church.[51] In 1673 in Dalkeith, Francis Scot, perhaps a man with powerful local kin, had been unable to persuade the session to let him buy himself off appearances, but was more effective at presbytery level, and there struck a bargain for one appearance only. In some places, for instance Ellon, Aberdeenshire, buying off penance had become regular in the 1750s, and in Foveran in the 1760s. Dalrymple session (Ayrshire) in 1769 made a ruling that anyone could avoid appearances by paying half a guinea; the fact that most offenders did not, and still faced public penance, shows that this level of payment was beyond their means. The practice became more general in the 1770s. A good example of the type of appeal comes in Straiton, Ayrshire, from 1778:

> Revd. Sir,
> This serves to inform you that Margaret Campbell my father's servant says she is with child and that it is mine. I think myself unlucky that I cannot deny the accusation and in order to give the church as little unnecessary trouble as in my power to do hereby acknowledge the charge. I am sorry for the offence given to God, I regret the injury done the poor Girl, and lament the breach of good order in society. I trust my future conduct will make it appear that my repentance is most sincere. I am ready to atone for the crime but am unwilling to make a public appearance which I hope your regulations will dispense with upon giving something to the poor.
> (sic subscrivitur) James Mcharg.

The session, delighted with the spirit of penitence, readily agreed.

The ability to write a smooth letter, and raise the money, meant that evasions of penance were more likely to be achieved by men than by women. Before the 1770s most sessions would not have responded, as did Straiton, to either, and indeed many felt uneasy with it. In the case quoted in Chapter 7 from Spott (1697), the minister was not happy that the offending man obtained remission of penance while the girl still had to do it. By contrast in Grange, 1771, an adulterer was let off penance on payment of 100 pounds Scots, while the woman made seven appearances.

If the opinion of some who managed church affairs had changed, parishioners still adhered to the rules. As Chapter 5 will show, there was little or no rise in illegitimacy ratios before 1780. Nor did men become less ready to admit their responsibility when named by the women (except in southern Scotland, and even then not much). In many parishes by the 1770s fornication cases, or antenuptial pregnancy instances, were brought to the sessions by couples coming forward voluntarily to report themselves. The absolution of the Church was still valued by those who had broken its rules and the practice of couples accepting being fined for fornication went on in some parishes until the end of the nineteenth century.[52]

Other elements in church discipline faded before the sexual. There was a decline in prosecutions for breach of sabbath observance from the 1740s, and the Church became less zealous over premarital pregnancy in the 1760s. So the weakening of discipline over fornication was the final stage. Action was still sometimes taken, but in the early nineteenth century private rebukes became more common. A traveller writing in 1807 spoke of the abandonment of public repentance by most ministers, for fear of causing child murder.[53] The relationship between Church and congregation had totally changed. By the 1770s it was no longer possible for the Church to keep up the old system of control. It was abandoned from the top while still acceptable to the bulk of the people.

Notes

1 S.G.E. Lythe, *The Economy of Scotland in its European Setting, 1550–1625* (Edinburgh, 1960), pp. 248–54.
2 Rosalind Mitchison, *Lordship to Patronage: Scotland 1603–1745* (London, 1983), p. 94.
3 W.R. Scott, *The Constitution of English, Scottish and Irish Joint Stock Companies* (London, 1912), vol. III, pp. 121–95.
4 *APS* VIII 595, IX 421. See Ian Whyte, *Agriculture and Society in Seventeenth-Century Scotland* (Edinburgh, 1979), Ch. 4.
5 R.A. Dodgshon, *Land and Society in Early Scotland* (Oxford, 1981), pp. 254–5, 281–4; Whyte, *Agriculture and Society*, pp. 192–4.
6 T.C. Smout, *A Century of the Scottish People, 1830–1950* (London, 1986), Ch. 3.
7 Bernard Bailyn, *Voyagers to the West* (London, 1987), Ch. 14.
8 Rosalind Mitchison, 'Patriotism and national identity in eighteenth-century Scotland', in T.W. Moody (ed.), *Nationality and the Pursuit of National Independence* (Belfast, 1978), pp. 85–8.
9 Christina Larner, 'Crimen Exceptum? The Crime of Witchcraft in Europe', in V.A.C. Gatrell, Bruce Lenman and Geoffrey Parker (eds.), *Crime and the Law* (London, 1980), pp. 68–71; Christina Larner, *Enemies of God* (London, 1981), Ch. 14.
10 John Burnett, *A Treatise on various branches of the Criminal Law of Scotland* (Edinburgh, 1811), p. 389; W.G. Scott-Moncrieff (ed.), *The Records of the proceedings of the Justiciary Court, Edinburgh, 1661–78* (Scottish History Society, Edinburgh, 1905), vol. 1, p. 196, vol. 2, p. xiv.
11 David Hume, *Commentaries on the law of Scotland respecting crimes* (Edinburgh, 1986), pp. 339–46.
12 C.H. Firth, *Scotland and the Protectorate* (Scottish History Society, Edinburgh, 1899), pp. 407–9; A. Fenton, *Scottish Country Life* (Edinburgh, 1976), pp. 52–6.
13 Rosalind Mitchison, *Life in Scotland* (London, 1978), pp. 67–8.
14 W.C. Hoskins, *The Midland Peasant* (London, 1957), Ch. 10; 'The Rebuilding of Rural England', *Provincial England* (London, 1963), pp. 131–48.

Girls in Trouble

15 E.g. the inventory of William McGuffog, SRO, Commissariot of Wigtown, 1705.
16 John Sinclair, *Analysis of the Statistical Account* (London, 1826), p. 244; L. Timperley, 'The pattern of landholding in eighteenth-century Scotland', in M.L. Parry and T.R. Slater (eds.), *The Making of the Scottish Countryside* (London, 1980), pp. 137–54.
17 Timperley, 'The pattern of landholding in eighteenth-century Scotland'.
18 This is clear from the biographical details in Hew Scott, *Fasti Ecclesiae Scoticanae,* 7 vols. (Edinburgh, 1915–28).
19 N.T. Phillipson and Rosalind Mitchison (eds.), *Scotland in the Age of Improvement* (Edinburgh, 1970).
20 *APS* viii 220, Act anent the poore (1649).
21 *APS* x 64, Act for the better provideing the Poor and repressing of Beggars (1696, confirmed 1701), in *APS* x Appendix 99b, Act anent the Poor.
22 Rosalind Mitchison, 'North and South: the development of the gulf in poor law practice', in R.A. Houston and Ian Whyte (eds.), *Scottish Society 1500–1800* (Cambridge, 1989), pp. 198–225.
23 Paton vs Adamson, in W. Wallace (ed.), *Decisions of the Court of Session for the Years 1772, 1773 and 1774* (Edinburgh, 1784).
24 Ian Whyte, *Agriculture and Society in Seventeenth-Century Scotland,* Ch. 4.
25 T.C. Smout, 'Where had the Scottish economy got to by the third quarter of the eighteenth century?', in Istvan Hunt and Michael Ignatieff (eds.), *Wealth and Virtue* (Cambridge, 1983), pp. 45–72.
26 J.G.A. Pocock, 'Cambridge paradigms and Scotch philosophers: a study of the relations between the civic humanist and the civil jurisprudential interpretation of eighteenth-century social thought', in ibid., p. 236.
27 NLS MS 6658, dated 1738 or 9, 'Essay on Female conduct'.
28 Richard B. Sher, *Church and University in the Scottish Enlightenment* (Edinburgh, 1985), Part 1.
29 *Ecclesiastical Characteristics* (1753) and *A Serious Apology for the Ecclesiastical Characteristics* (Edinburgh, 1763).
30 Hugh Arnot, *A Collection and Abridgement of Celebrated Criminal Trials in Scotland from AD 1536 to 1784* (Edinburgh, 1785), pp. 322–7.
31 State Papers, Ireland, Letters and Papers, PRO SP 63/364, anonymous letter from Edinburgh, 19 November 1704, to Edward Southwell, Dublin. We thank T.C. Smout for this reference.
32 N. Morren, *Annals of the General Assembly of the Church of Scotland* (Edinburgh, 1838), vol. 1, pp. 158–67, 280.
33 Rosalind Mitchison, 'The Making of the Old Scottish Poor Law', *Past and Present 63* (1974), pp. 58–93.
34 D. Withrington, 'Non-Church Going, *c.*1750–*c.*1850: A Preliminary Study', *Records of the Scottish Church History Society* xvii (1972), pp. 91–113.
35 Patrick Bannerman, *Sermon upon Reformation and Revolution Principles preached in the Church of Stirling April 10 1751 by appointment of the Synod* (Edinburgh, 1751), pp. 19–20; James Oswald, *Sermon at the opening of the General Assembly May 1766, to which are annexed Letters* (Edinburgh, 1766), p. 29; OSA vi (1793), p. 609, Appendix, 'Letters addressed to Sir John Sinclair by William Creech'.
36 Andrew L. Drummond and James Bulloch, *The Scottish Church 1688–1843* (Edinburgh, 1973), pp. 35–44; W. Ferguson, *Scotland, 1689 to the Present* (Edinburgh, 1968), pp. 118–23.
37 Arthur Fawcett, *The Cambuslang Revival* (London, 1971); T.C. Smout, 'Born again at Cambuslang: new evidence on popular religion and literacy in eighteenth century Scotland', *Past and Present 97* (1982), pp. 114–27.
38 The figure is quoted in Bruce Lenman, *Integration, Enlightenment and Industrialisation: Scotland 1746–1832* (London, 1981), p. 146.

2: The Changing Economic and Social Setting

39 Norah Smith, 'Robert Wallace's "Of Venery"', *Texas Studies in Literature and Language* *15* (1973), pp. 429–44.
40 Richard B. Sher, *Church and University*, Ch. 3.
41 *OSA* xvi (1795), Inveresk, pp. 1–52.
42 *Scots Magazine*, February 1757, pp. 80–2, and August 1757, pp. 401–2.
43 This Act, not surprisingly, was presented by the Reverend William Auld to the congregation of Mauchline parish, and is set out in the KSR of the parish.
44 The anonymous author was Dugald Graham.
45 *Records of the Most Ancient and Puissant Order of the Beggar's Benison and Merryland* (privately printed in Anstruther, 1892). This organisation and the fashion for overt sexual references among the upper classes are discussed in Norah Smith, 'Sexual mores and attitudes in Enlightenment Scotland', in P.C. Boucé (ed.), *Sexuality in Eighteenth-Century Britain* (Manchester, 1982), pp. 47–73. The SRO collections in which the Beggar's Benison are mentioned are Leven and Melville (GD 26) Dalguise (GD 38) Airlie (GD 16) and Dalhousie (GD 45). These are all early deposits, represented in the first printed volume of catalogue for GD (Gifts and Deposits). There may well have been more acquired later.
46 That this new attitude was not confined to Scotland is indicated by the changing response of the Roman Catholic clergy in the diocese of Montauban, southern France, to requests for dispensations for marriages within the prohibited degrees. After 1770 these clerics displayed a new readiness to admit the validity of affection as grounds for dispensation. Margaret H. Darrow, 'Popular concepts of marital choice in eighteenth century France', *Journal of Social History 19* (1985–6), pp. 261–72. A similar change is shown by the prison reform initiative of John Howard in England; and by the general failure in England to impose the death penalty for relatively minor offences. L. Radinowicz, *A History of English Criminal Law*, vol. 1 (London, 1948), Chs. 3, 4, 5. There was also the failure to apply penalties to the increasing number of people with Unitarian beliefs, a form of dissent not covered by the Toleration Act of 1690, and the new anti-slave trade movement.
47 *Scots Magazine*, 1780, pp. 238–41.
48 Maurice Lindsay, *Robert Burns* (London, 1954), p. 77.
49 K. Boyd, *Scottish Church Attitudes to Sex, Marriage and the Family* (Edinburgh, 1980).
50 Ian Whyte has made a special study of the process of urbanisation in Scotland which shows that the urban sector there grew more rapidly in the eighteenth century than in any other European country, and that much of the growth was in the small towns. See Ian D. Whyte, *Scotland before the Industrial Revolution* (London, 1995), Chs. 10, 11.
51 W. Cramond and S. Ree (eds.), *The Records of Elgin*, vol. 2 (New Spalding Club, Aberdeen, 1908), p. 4.
52 Cases can frequently be found in KSRs. See also Boyd, *Scottish Church Attitudes*, Chs. 3 and 9.
53 Boyd, *Scottish Church Attitudes*, Ch. 2; James Hall, *Travels in Scotland* (London, 1807), vol. ii, p. 351.

3

Regular Marriage

Before we can discuss the bearing of children out of wedlock, it is essential first to establish what actually constituted wedlock, a question by no means as straightforward as it might appear. Scots law allowed for the legitimation of children by the subsequent marriage of their parents, but in this enquiry we are concerned only with the status of children at birth. In any case such legitimation was relevant only to those owning property.

The first part of this chapter looks at the definition of marriage mainly from the viewpoint of the law and the higher courts, both civil and ecclesiastical. The second part looks at the line taken by kirk sessions.

Post-Reformation Scotland adhered on marriage to what a modern historian has called a 'blindingly simple doctrine' and a nineteenth-century English judge labelled 'monstrous' and 'barbarous', that if two people capable of marriage freely declared that they married each other, this constituted a valid marriage.[1] Marriage was not a sacrament: in the *Westminster Directory,* the usual service book for Scotland, it was made clear that the minister declared a couple married because they had given their mutual consents. The bars to marriage were few. The couple had to be free of any current marriage, they had to be capable of intercourse and of age (fourteen for boys and twelve for girls), and they must not be within the prohibited degrees of kindred or affinity.

Church and State agreed on how marriage should be conducted. Regular marriage consisted of the proclamation of banns in the parish churches of the couple on three consecutive Sundays, followed by exchange of consents in the church 'in the face of the congregation'. The parish would extract a deposit, known as 'consignation money', at the time of proclamation as a guarantee of behaviour. It would eventually be returned to the couple, unless there had been an undue amount of merrymaking at the wedding or the first child was born too soon for conception to have taken place within marriage. Session material does not expand on the particular forms of popular ritual and joviality which it aimed at repressing. A phrase used to cover unseemly wedding celebrations was 'penny weddings': these were forbidden as boisterous and likely to involve scandalous carriage and drunkenness. Church and State in the seventeenth century were united in disapproving of these affairs, though for different reasons. The State tried to prevent large assemblies of people where feuds might originate, and tried to limit the number of attenders at all rites of passage: weddings were particularly the subject of prohibitions by Parliament and the Privy Council in the 1680s. The Church's disapproval was made known by rulings of the lesser courts, sometimes in conjunction with burgh councils.[2]

There is some evidence that by the later eighteenth century the three proclamations might be made all on the same day. At various times the General Assembly or a presbytery had ruled on what days and parts of days the celebration of marriage should take place: the *First Book of Discipline,* for instance, required it to be on a Sunday and before noon, whereas later the Church tried to keep marriage off either Sunday or Saturday because the sabbath might be defaced by unsuitable merrymaking afterwards. Andrew Symson, for Galloway in the late seventeenth century, says that almost all marriages in his church had taken place on a Tuesday or a Thursday and while the moon was waxing,[3] but there seems to have been no ecclesiastical ruling on this.

Where a couple was free to marry the essential requirement was consent. Consent, the 'one thing sufficient and indispensable' for marriage, in the eyes of both Church and State, had to be free, that is, not the result of force, fraud or frivolity. In the later years of James VI the Privy Council had been much concerned with problems of abduction and rape, and had produced an Act of 1612 against ravishers of women, but its main motive was not so much the woman's own consent as the prevention of seductions and marriages which went against the wishes of parents. In 1688 it annulled marriage between a young girl and her music teacher in which a witness had been in disguise, and put the teacher in the pillory.[4]

The Church seems to have been uncertain about the dividing line between deception and persuasion. In 1729 the Reverend Robert Wodrow wrote out a long debate with himself over a case in which a girl of thirteen had been beguiled into marriage with the 23 year old son of her foster parents, under the impression that he would otherwise die. In spite of the fact that the girl had no idea of the significance of marriage promises, and that the Church at various times had stated that knowledge of the Christian religion and of the mutual duties of husband and wife should be ascertained before a marriage took place, Wodrow did not appear to consider that the marriage could be declared invalid.[5]

The issue of parental consent was one where Church and State diverged in the seventeenth century. The *Directory* of 1645 required anyone under 21 to request the consent of parents before a marriage was proclaimed. In 1644 the General Assembly had considered a motion which would have enabled the propertied parents of boys under 21 to invalidate betrothals which followed fornication with women whose friends were stated to have 'seduced' the young boys into promises. The language of the motion was heavily slanted against the women. We do not know if the motion was passed, but it ran counter to the views of the Church on the basis of marriage in free consent. In 1646, for instance, the Synod of Lothian and Tweeddale told the presbytery of Dunbar that it should attempt to obtain parental consent in cases where there had already been intercourse 'under promises'. The editor of the records of this synod holds that this shows that parental consent was 'virtually essential', but the evidence does not show that it was regarded as more than desirable.[6] This had been the stance taken by the Church in the *First Book of Discipline,* and remained so in the early eighteenth century. Parental consent was desirable and should not be withheld for worldly reasons. A couple with a recalcitrant parent would be urged to be considerate, but it is clear from instances given below that there was no real obstacle to marriage against the wishes of parents. Unhappy parents would have to use other sanctions, like the couple who in 1758 advertised in an Edinburgh newspaper that their children, if marrying against parental wishes, would be disinherited.[7]

Parental consent came up in the lay courts or the Privy Council only when there was property involved. Cases in the later seventeenth century, all based on the

Border region, show that in any disagreement between mother and father over a match, it was the father's views that counted. In the Ayton case of 1678, when one part of the Home kinship wished to secure a Home heiress, the girl was abducted as soon as she reached the age of twelve and married to the juvenile George Home in England. Fines were imposed for contempt of Council, to whom the control of the girl had been given, and for contempt of the Church by a marriage by an English minister, but the marriage was not declared invalid.[8]

Parental consent will be discussed further when we look at kirk session material, but it is clear that for unpropertied couples the main obstacle which prevented sexual union being confirmed by formal marriage was, as elsewhere in Western Europe, the accepted need of a couple to be able to support a family. What scraps of information we have on the age of marriage in Scotland and the proportion not marrying imply that the European pattern of late and restricted marriage opportunities operated here also.[9] For marriage to be feasible a man needed a secure slot in the economy, as a tenant or a cottar in peasant society, or as a craftsman. But most young adults were insecure, working as servants or apprentices and living in the households of their masters, and not in a position to marry.

The Church barred any marriage that it considered incestuous, where the couple were within the prohibited degrees of kindred or affinity. These were defined in Leviticus XVIII, and confirmed by legislation,[10] as parents, siblings, aunts and uncles, children and grandchildren, and half-siblings; plus their spouses and equivalents by marriage. A genealogist would call such kin first and second degrees of kin; first cousins are only related in the third degree and could marry.

A taboo against incest is long-standing in western society. We do not know why the Reformed Church continued to be so concerned about incest, but it was not based on any fear of inbreeding or defective offspring. Calvin's assertion that the Old Testament was as authoritative as the New doubtless influenced the Scottish Church. The 1690 Confession of Faith asserted that 'a man may not marry any of his wife's kindred nearer in blood than he may of his own, nor the woman any of her husband's kindred nearer in blood than of her own.'[11] And the Church was always concerned with the stability of marriage and may have realised that if sexual overtures and rivalries were allowed to develop within the close family, that family would quickly be torn apart. From this viewpoint the links of affinity – those created by marriage – were just as important as those arising from blood.

The legislation of 1690 was a definition of affinity solely in relationship to marriage, but the Church introduced to this the concept of affinity by sexual intercourse. In Blair Atholl, in December 1751, Katharine Stewart's proclamation of marriage with John Gow was stopped following an allegation of indecent behaviour with Alexander Gow, his brother. When Alexander admitted the fornication, the proposed marriage was called incestuous and banned. In a case of the preceding century (Pencaitland, March 1666), a mere allegation of scandalous carriage between a man and a girl some years before was enough to lead the session to block his proposed marriage to her sister on the grounds of possible incest. Agnes McLaren in Kenmore (December 1755) was in trouble over an affair with the man married to her sister, but since the affair preceded the contract of marriage it was not called incest. In 1768 in New Monkland the session refused marriage to Helen Wilkie and Duncan Shaw on evidence of what would now be called 'petting' between her and his brother some seven years earlier. The witness of these activities had been a girl of twelve at the time, but 'it was the received opinion of the neighbourhood that they would marry.' The session stated that the evidence was not sufficient for a legal process. It also said that, if ordered by a superior court, it would allow the marriage.

According to Leviticus XVIII affinity by marriage was removed by death, but the Church did not hold this view, and the State, which regarded incest as a capital offence, apparently concurred. In the 1705 case of William Drysdale and Barbara Tannahill the man had intercourse with his deceased wife's sister. Tannahill confessed and was executed, Drysdale denied the charge and was banished. Some time after this, legal opinion seemed to favour staying within the precise wording of Leviticus XVIII, though in an annulment case of 1825 the marriage of a man with his brother's widow was considered illegal and invalid.[12] But, as with other matters, the law had by then relaxed its severity, and the absence of incest trials suggests that there was little legal enthusiasm for such matters.

Marriage was for life; however, very soon after the Reformation the Church declared that divorce was available in cases of adultery. (Between 1560 and 1563, when a national consistory court was set up in Edinburgh, divorces were handled by kirk sessions.) The biblical penalty for adultery was death, a penalty which the reformers would have liked to see rigorously applied. The secular compromise was to have the guilty party declared legally dead, with all the financial consequences that entailed, and the innocent party was free to remarry.[13] There remained the problem of whether the adulterer, if he was not to be executed, could remarry, and, in particular, whether he could marry his paramour. The Church's belief that marriage was necessary to prevent sin led to acceptance of the right to remarriage, but in 1601 an Act of Parliament forbade marriage to the paramour.[14]

Divorce for adultery was a genuine possibility for anyone who could afford to go to court. But, at least in the seventeenth century, the guilty party was at risk of criminal conviction for 'notour' or persistent adultery, and this carried the death penalty. Nevertheless, the wording of the relevant Act of 1581 appears designed to make conviction unlikely. 'Notour' adultery had to involve open and persistent cohabitation, continuing after warnings and excommunication. The few adulterers sentenced to death were all exceptionally flagrant offenders, and seem to have been victims of the seventeenth-century tendency to stretch the criminal law against offenders considered generally undesirable. Even in the 1670s more usual was banishment, whipping, fine or prison. As late as 1699 a couple was banished, but clearly the Act of 1581 was not being fully used.[15]

Divorce for desertion was more slowly established. An Act of Parliament of 1573 stated that after four years of desertion without reasonable cause, proved in front of a judge, a deserted spouse could sue for 'adherence', that is return of the deserter, in the Commissary Court. If this did not produce a return, the spouse could obtain letters 'of four Forms', later letters of horning, in the Court of Session.[16] The deserter could then be called on by the bishop to adhere, and be excommunicated if this failed. Divorce was then achieved. Attempts in the 1690s to get the procedure simplified failed, and the law stood thus, with replacement of the action by the bishop with action by a presbytery, until the 1860s.

It was not necessary to trace the spouse who had deserted in order to instigate a divorce action on that ground: the name of the missing person would be called out at the market square of Edinburgh and pier and shore of Leith, and if there was no response the process would go ahead in his or her absence. It was even possible to

Girls in Trouble

bring a case 'under benefit of the poors' roll' if one did not have the means to do so otherwise, but in rural Scotland in our period no one even thought of doing such a thing; it was not part of the culture.

This meant that a man or woman who had been deserted and wanted to remarry would have to try and ascertain if the deserter was still alive or not. Men or women who deserted were unlikely to set up house where they could be traced by kirk sessions; they simply walked away from family responsibilities, sometimes to England, sometimes to become a soldier if male, or to cohabit with one if female, leaving no trace. The sessions dealing with the wish of a deserted person to remarry would require evidence of the death of the first spouse. The couple would have to advertise for the missing spouse at the ports, or to trace witnesses to his or her death. All this cost time and money. In June 1717 Helen Roberts in Torphichen, a deserted wife, admitted that she was pregnant by a man Thomson. 'Being asked if her Husband was dead she answered she knew not Only she was informed by One that was in the Ship with him that he dyed in the Ship going to Flanders And told she never heard from him since he went Away which was nine years since'. She was forbidden to have private converse with Thomson and the case, which would be one of adultery if her husband was still alive, was referred to the presbytery. A year later she and Thomson were ordered to be rebuked, so it appears that they got off lightly. Sessions would accept hearsay evidence of a death, and long silence after public enquiries at ports might count towards a presumption of death. In Stranraer in 1698 three years disappearance and a search of seaports allowed the session to consider a husband's death morally certain. A woman in Pencaitland (October 1701), whose husband had disappeared in a nearby parish which was overwhelmed by deaths in the famine of the 1690s, was helped by the minister to advertise for him, and had her liaison treated as mere fornication.

Although the only court that could ultimately pronounce on the legality or dissolution of a marriage was Edinburgh Commissary Court, in our period it was chiefly the propertied who would have recourse to that court. At the level of small tenants, subtenants and cottars, it was the kirk session who would first be referred to on marriage questions. Apart from its disciplinary function, the session was frequently called upon – especially in the seventeenth and early eighteenth century – to act as mediator in local disputes and disagreements, and therefore it is not surprising to find it intervening in matters concerning marriage. Thus, by means of kirk session records, we are enabled to move from legislation and broad theoretical views on marriage to specific local examples of how various aspects of marriage were regarded and treated at parish level.

The first stage was the promise of marriage. As will be seen in the next chapter, the importance of this was that under civil law a promise of marriage followed by sexual intercourse constituted a legal marriage. But such promises were rarely witnessed and difficult to prove. An unmarried woman who became pregnant might claim that this was under promise of marriage, but this would not get her very far unless the man concurred. In Eskdalemuir (February 1753) Jean Linton claimed that the man responsible, who was the church precentor, had promised her marriage. His response was that he had made proposals of marriage but no solemn promise. He lost his church position because of the scandal but was not considered under an obligation to marry her. Even when a man admitted the promise he still might not fulfil it. In Troqueer (April 1759) Isabell McGarroch named John Ogilvie, who had recently admitted being responsible for another woman's pregnancy, as father of her unborn child. She claimed he had often promised to marry her, 'both before and after his guilt with her'. He 'acknowledged that he told the said Isabell that he intended to marry her and added that he continued in that intention till about a Month ago, when he received some Informations which made him alter his design of Marriage'. No further light is thrown on the nature of his objection, and he was exhorted to fulfil his intention of marriage with her 'as the best Reparation he could make her for seducing her to be guilty with him'. Whether he actually did so is not known.

The question of promise of marriage surfaces most frequently in cases where a woman attempted to stop a marriage proclamation on the grounds that a promise had previously been made to her. Kirk sessions took such allegations seriously. In Kilmarnock (June 1699) Isobel Robertson voluntarily confessed to fornication in order to stop the man's marriage to someone else. The man denied promises of marriage to her, but the session stopped his marriage proclamations with the other woman until the alleged promise was investigated. In Kilbrandon (March 1759) Ann McDougald, on hearing that Alan Campbell was about to marry another woman, came to the session to stop the proclamations, presenting to them 'four letters from the said Alan containing the strongest protestations of Love & most solemn promises of Marriage within a month or six weeks time that possibly could be.' She also declared she was with child to him, which he did not deny. 'But he refused to adhere to his former promises of Marriage to her & declared that he would never marry her upon any account.' The session ordered his proclamations with the other woman to be stopped and 'desired Ann McDougald if she had a mind that she might pursue Alan as Law would direct'.

In some cases, the session realised that the woman was not really expecting to stop a marriage but had a more mercenary motive. Two such cases appeared in the same year in Drainie (April and November 1708), and a note of cynicism is evident in the records. In the first one Ann Gordon attempted to stop the marriage of James Cuming to another woman. Cuming denied having given her any promise and said he could swear to this:

> The Session alledging they had grounds enough to suspect he could not swear so, with a good conscience, as also supposing that if he gave the forsaid Ann a piece of money (which was all she was aiming at) she would pass from her compearance. They advised the said James that it would be every way his safest course to give so much to the said Ann, as would satisffie her, whither he had made any promises to her or not.

Cuming refused to pay her, and eventually the session agreed to give her 20 merks 'for paying her penalty & nursing his child', and allowed the proclamations to proceed.

In the second case, Christian Ritchie, who had had William Winster's child, wanted to stop his marriage proclamations. As far as the session were concerned, 'it was not so much marriage as a piece of money the Woman aimed at.' The man denied promising to marry her, 'and said if he gave her any money to silence her clamours, it would not be so much as she would demand.' Once again the proclamations were temporarily stopped, but he gave her some money in the end.

More unusually, in Kilmarnock (November 1742) a man complained against a woman. John Campbell said he had had repeated promises of marriage from Mary

Girls in Trouble

McKissag, as well as the consent of her mother and stepfather, but that she was now proclaimed with another man. He craved the session 'wou'd oblige her to adhere to her first Promises or see the Complainer have justice as to the Expence incurrd by him in his Courtship.' Mary McKissag admitted 'she was so foolish as to make & give several Promises to the said John to that Effect but they were only on Condition that all her Friends [i.e. relatives] would be satisfyd with the Match and confessed she was once willing to marry the said John but found her friends against it.' Her mother agreed that 'she was witness to several Promises which passd between them & for her part was not against the Match but she found her Daughters friends were rather inclin'd she shou'd marry the Person to whom she is now contracted.' The session found Mary McKissag to blame 'for her rash Promises', but as she repented and had been contracted and proclaimed with the second man, her marriage was allowed to proceed. Campbell was told to apply to the civil magistrate 'in Regard the Session can do nothing as to his Expences.'

A most interesting case concerning promise of marriage arose in Kinglassie (April 1760). The church's precentor reported that after George Chrystie, foreman to the Earl of Rothes, had been proclaimed for the first time with Janet Storrar, a widow, Ann Robertson had put in his hands a formal Protest, on the grounds that Chrystie had given her promises of marriage both before and after the birth of their illegitimate child six years earlier. Subsequently she had put in his hands a Discharge, 'loosing the said George from any promise of marriage she had asserted he had given her for the sum of four pound sterling he had paid to her in order to be loosed from said Promises and allowing him to go on with the proclamation.' However, in the Discharge she still insisted there had been repeated promises of marriage, and because of this some doubt had arisen about the legality of Chrystie's proposed marriage with Janet Storrar. Ann Robertson was called before the session and reiterated the claim, declaring 'that she reckoned herself married to him till Death should part them tho' she was not to pursue him if he married another.' She had nothing to gain by making such a statement, and presumably sincerely believed that even if Chrystie married someone else his promise to her had been equivalent to a marriage vow. The fact that this promise alone – even after she had released him from it – gave cause for doubt concerning the legality of another marriage (though, as Ann Robertson raised no further claims on him, he was eventually allowed to proceed) shows that the Church could at times take a promise of marriage as seriously as a contract. More seriously, even, for there are a number of breaches of marriage contracts in our records, and they rarely created as much consternation as the above case.[17]

The contract was the stage following promise of marriage and preceding proclamation of banns. In Dundee (February 1691), Andrew Jameson confessed fornication with Katharine Creightoune and did not deny it was under promise of marriage, 'but he says he was willing to Contract with hir befor the scandall brok out but she would not therefor he is free of his promise.' The woman acknowledged that he had 'offered to contract with her befor the scandal brok out but she says she desyred him to delay it for a day till she payd off some small debts she was resting (owing) that he might not say he had maried ane woman drownd in debt and so render the rest of her lyff comfortless.' (This is one of a number of cases we found where seventeenth- and eighteenth-century women demonstrated their independence.) The minister subsequently persuaded Jameson 'to perform his promise of marriage to hir'.

46

3: Regular Marriage

There is some indication in the material on fornication before marriage (see Chapter 5) that some couples regarded the contract as equivalent to the later marriage ceremony and went to bed together on the strength of it. Needless to say, the Church did not concur with this view. However, 'resiling' from a marriage contract was not very difficult, although a hefty fine would normally be exacted. Various reasons were given for resiling. When Canisbay session (January 1729) asked Isobell Rigg why she had stopped the proclamation of banns with Magnus McBeath she replied that,

> prior to her Contracting with him he gave himself out for more substance than he really had, & That he had no settled Residence, so that after their Marriage they would be oblig'd to go to service & that she chooses rather to keep in service while she is single than be oblig'd to serve when ty'd in Wedlock.

Mary Couper in Thurso (December 1727) said the man responsible for her pregnancy had contracted to marry her but now refused. He said this was because 'there were some things promised to him by her friends antecedent to the Marriage which were not performed.'

Kirk sessions would consider any reasonable grounds for not going on with a marriage; what they objected strongly to was 'flighty' behaviour. In Canisbay (January 1713) Jean Grott had broken marriage contracts with two men and laid the blame on them. One of the men was asked why he resiled and replied that it was the woman's doing; 'being interrogate if he was still willing to marry her, Answer'd he found her ane unsettl'd changable woman.' The session declared Jean Grott to be 'a foolish unsolid woman' who should be severely fined. Also in Canisbay (February 1730) Donald Banks, when asked why he stopped his proclamation of marriage with Barbara Mcferson, 'said his Heart did not lie to it Being asked if he had any further Objection said he had none Whereupon the Session taking his Inconstancy and Perfidiousness to Consideration appoint the Session Baillie to Decern him in a fine of ten pound Scots.'

One must assume in the above case that the session believed the man was taking the matter altogether too lightly; reasons of lack of inclination or incompatibility were listened to sympathetically. Two such cases appeared in Kilmory session records. In August 1707 Elizabeth NcGrigor's father brought a complaint against James Stuart for resiling from his contract with her. Stuart explained that,

> his mind & inclination did not at all from first to last sway that way although in a manner compelled to tender love to the said Elizabeth NcGrigor through the continuall importunity of his friends and relations who in some measure contrary to his own will contracted them together. Moreover he added that he never had true affection for her.

The session declared they 'truly think him under no obligation to marry the said person especially considering that... the said Elizabeth NcGrigor did freely quitt with him, allowing him his freedom of choice in his marriage with any other he pleased.'

This attitude was made even plainer in an earlier case (August 1704). John Fergusson, when asked why he resiled from marrying Margaret NcMurchie, 'told that he had no other reason than this, that his Inclination did not tend that way & therefore could not marry her without the greatest reluctancy In regard he had no true

Girls in Trouble

love for her.' Being asked 'what moved him to proceed so farr on in a matter of this moment, Replyed, that it was the advice of his Friends, rather than his own Choice & Inclination.' After debating the matter, the session 'considering the Inconveniences that might follow upon the Restraint & Compulltion of the Session in a matter of free choice which ought to be carried on from a principal of Love and affection between parties Contracted in Order to a married state thought fit to leave him to his own minde, only forfeiting the Consignation money from him.'

As has been indicated, parents' consent was not a legal requirement for adults to marry, though we have seen that pressure by parents and relatives influenced the choice of partner. In Foveran (October 1736) a letter from Mary Young was laid before the session in which she stated that, although she had been proclaimed the previous Sunday with John Milne, 'it is evidently known to God & the world that I hade no design to marry him, only to satisfy my Parents.' She went on to ask to be proclaimed with the man of her own choice, Alexander Aberdeen. There was also a letter from John Milne entreating that the proclamations be continued. However, the session clerk advised that Mary Young's father had desired the proclamations be stopped, and the woman herself appearing before the session with Alexander Aberdeen, 'judicially declared their mutual adherence to one another and craved of the Session to be three times proclaimed this day in order to marriage. Upon all which the Session finding it was too Evident the said Mary hade been compelled to give consent to the said John Milne, did agree their proclamations should be intimate.'

The parental pressure in that case was in favour of a particular partner; more usual was parental opposition. In Sorn (September 1723) Margaret White and James Wilson had three illegitimate children before they finally married, the delay being 'because of his fathers great aversion'. In Pencaitland (December 1711), when Christian Bennet gave birth to an illegitimate child in secret, it was said that the reason for this was that the man had uttered threats, 'he being affraid of his mother, who had hindered him to marry the said Christian Bennet.'

In Calder (July 1699), a girl's father objected to her chosen marriage partner. He was not able to give any grounds for his opposition but said to the minister, 'he might marrie them if he liked but he should leave his blood upon them and him that married these.' The couple were given permission to marry but admonished to deal calmly and tenderly with the parent. John Leckie and Janet Futt (Fossoway, February 1718) asked to be proclaimed, but the session, being informed that the girl's parents objected to the man, insisted on hearing the reasons first, which were given as follows:

> 1mo in regard he never countenanced her parents in the matter 2do that he unsuitably inticed her out of her parents house both in the night and day time without their knowledge 3tio that the match is altogether unequal in respect of parentage 4to & ultimo that he never proposed any manner of way for her to live suitable to her fathers Daughter.

None of these reasons gave just grounds to stop the marriage going forward.

The two main reasons for parental opposition were economic circumstances and supposed inequalities of status. In Dysart (April 1671) the session allowed the marriage of David Anderson and Euphan Marton to go ahead in spite of her mother's opposition, 'the Session finding, after they had heard her, that shee asserts nothing against the young man, except as shee alledges, that his state is not so good as shee wold have it.' In Sorn (November 1707) James Brown's father objected to his son's proposed marriage to Margaret Smith 'because as he thinks of its inconveniency by reason of the mean poor circumstances of both parties'; the proclamations were allowed to proceed.

As parental opposition without genuine legal grounds was not sufficient to stop a marriage, it is not surprising that the sessions in those cases reached the decisions they did. In the two instances where we found sessions having problems, it was not because more valid objections were made but because the parties involved were of higher social standing. In a Wigtown case (September 1719) Provost Gulline, a church elder, wanted to marry Jean McKie, daughter of a landowner, David McKie of Maidland. Maidland opposed the marriage, and as he was going to be away asked the session to decide nothing in his absence. The session asked the provost to do everything in his power to obtain Maidland's consent, but it seems he was not successful, for when they met again Maidland was still opposing the marriage. It is clear that the reasons he put forward were not sufficient, for the marriage was allowed, but the session deferred sufficiently to the landowner to impose special conditions, that the contract of marriage would be drawn up in the sight of someone whom Maidland would appoint and then be deposited with the minister or a member of the session. The provost expressed indignation at such treatment, 'whereupon the Session declare that they find it agreeable to the discipline of the Church of Scotland and the Word of God that all caution and deliberation be exercised by the judicatories of the Church, especially when parents refuse their consent upon reasons to the marriage of their children.' Such caution and deliberation did not appear so necessary to kirk sessions when members of the gentry class were not involved.

The other gentry case we found occurred in Belhelvie (March 1729), when John Montfod, officer of excise, applied for proclamation of banns to Susana Ker, daughter to Alexander Ker of Meny. The minister was 'straitned and difficulted in this matter on account of Meny and his Lady their refusal to give their Consent'. The session advised Montfod that they could proceed no further at the time, 'upon which he represented to the Session that Parents their refusall to consent to the Mariage of their Children, is not sufficient to hinder the proclamation of their Matrimoniall banns, unless they give clear and convincing reasons, for their dissent, which he said, Meny and his Lady had not done in this case.' The session continued to procrastinate, and an angry Montfod appealed to presbytery. Legally the session did not have a leg to stand on, but it is clear it was thoroughly cowed by this local landowner.

We found only one case where the session acted to stop a marriage opposed by a parent, and the son concerned in that case was a minor (Kilmory, August 1704). Even then the session did not simply forbid the marriage, as legally it might have done. It called the couple before it and asked if they had promised to marry one another, to which they both replied that they had:

> The Session therefor taking occasion from their Confessions to represent to them both, the folly, the rashness, hazerd & inconveniences, together with the bad Consequences of suchlike irreligious & irrational promises how sinfull they are in the sight of God, and even the invalidity of their Promise in parlar is in the sight of man especially when done in their Minority and nonage, and how grievous it might prove to their parants, and other friends or well-wishers of their concerns, and especially when so Repugnant to the Doctrine of the Gospell, as incroaching upon

> the most holy & wise Providence of the soverraigne Disposer of all Creatures and in all their actions and that notwithstanding of their Proposing yet God would dispose as he thought fit and conveneint for them, thus the Vanity of their foolish promise being Represented to them.

Given this storm of reproach the youngsters capitulated and agreed to part.

The concern of kirk sessions with marriage did not end with the ceremony. There are cases throughout our period of sessions intervening as what might now be termed marriage counsellors. In Dailly (April 1694) the session cited James Davisone and Janet McClure, his wife, for not living together. The man 'says it is not his fault for he is content to live with her, Janet McClure compeirs and says that she cannot have a heart to live with her husband at all, she is rebuked & commanded to live with her husband under the pain of being prosecuted for wilful desertion.' In other words, affection might be important in determining the marriage partner, but once married a woman had made her bed and must lie on it.

The attitude expressed in the above case towards a woman unhappy in her marriage is echoed constantly during our period. All the other cases we collected involved men actually ill-treating their wives, yet in none of them did the session consider this justify the wife leaving her husband. At least in the seventeenth century the session might impose financial constraints on the man to make him behave better. In Grange (May 1684) Alexander Gawin and his wife were cited before the session for their 'Unchristian & unconjugall way of living, he by oppressing & striking of her, especiallie on the Sabbath day, & she by deserting of him, & not cohabiting with him, he was enjoined to find surety that she should be harmless & skaithlesse of him (as also her children) in all tyme coming.' In another seventeenth-century case (Sorn, November 1697) the woman said she would only return to her husband if 'he find cautione for her life & fortune'. The session declined to take this on themselves but advised her, 'if she would have him obliedged so to do, she behoved to get him obliedged befor a judge.'

In the late seventeenth century sessions frequently intervened against wife beating, and not only when it took place on the sabbath or caused public scandal (for instance by the wife taking refuge in the house of another family). This suggests that there was, for a period, a real attempt to curb domestic violence. In the eighteenth century cases are less frequent, but it is not clear whether this is because the attempt had been abandoned, or because violence had lessened.

In the eighteenth century sessions appeared to consider a promise of good behaviour in cases of marital violence sufficient without legal obligations. In Canisbay (August 1729) it was reported that Andrew Groat and Katharine Lyell were living apart. He,

> being Interrogate why he put away his Wife said he did what in him lay to persuade her to stay with him but she would not. The said Katharine Lyell being Interrogate why she would not Cohabite with her Husband said she was afraid of her Life if she would stay with him Being asked if he did strick her at any time said he did not but threatened her oft times & he hounded out his sister-in-law to abuse & threaten her & she accordingly came to the House & did so. The said Andrew Groat being asked if he would accept of his Wife again said he would wherupon being Exhorted to be more loving & tender of her than formerly & set up the Worship of God in his Family & she being Exhorted to be more obedient.

3: Regular Marriage

The sting in the tail of those last words shows how the Church viewed a woman's role in a marriage.

By the second half of the eighteenth century sessions were unlikely to intervene even if they knew a married couple was not cohabiting. However, in Kenmore (June 1755) a woman brought her own case before the session. Florence McGrigor complained that her husband, Donald McGrigor, 'us'd her barbarously for these four years past, and that she is not able to bear with the bad usage she meets from him and declares that if he does not treat her better she'll be obliged to part with him, therefore begg'd the session to do what they can to redress her grievances.' The husband, when cited, 'compear'd professing his sorrow for what differences had happened betwixt him and his wife, and promises that, God assisting, he shall so behave towards her as becomes a husband to his wife; And she promises that she shall be dutiful as becomes a wife.' The final exhortation comes as no surprise by now, and one can hardly avoid being sceptical of the promises of a man who had ill-treated his wife for four years, but at least in the changing climate of the time, the kirk session was less likely to interfere if she did in the end go off and leave him.

In its approach to marital disharmony the Kirk did not discriminate between couples married regularly and those with irregular marriages. The emphasis on consent meant that marriage was marriage however arrived at. The ramifications of irregular marriage form the subject of our next chapter.

Notes

1 T.C. Smout, 'Scottish Marriage, Regular and Irregular, 1500–1940', in R.B. Outhwaite (ed.), *Marriage and Society* (London, 1981), pp. 204–36; *Report of the Select Committee on the marriage law, Scotland* (PP 1849 xii), p. 15, Mr Baron Bayley, quoted by Lord Brougham.
2 Henry Grey Graham, *Social Life in Scotland in the Eighteenth Century* (London, 1937), p. 186; J.R. Hardy, 'The Attitudes of Church and State in Scotland to Sex and Marriage, 1500–1707' (unpublished M.Phil. thesis, Edinburgh University, 1978), Ch. 4; *RPCS* viii, p. 496 (1684), and XIII, p. viii (1687), *APS* viii 350 (1681).
3 Andrew Symson, *A Large Description of Galloway* (Edinburgh, 1823), p. 95.
4 *RPCS* xiii, p. 207 (1688), Sir John Lauder of Fountainhall, *Historical Notices* (Bannatyne Club, Edinburgh, 1848), II, p. 858.
5 Robert Wodrow, *Analecta* (Maitland Club, Edinburgh, 1843), IV, p. 33.
6 James Kirk (ed.), *The Records of the Synod of Lothian and Tweeddale* (Stair Society, Edinburgh, 1977), pp. xiv, 191.
7 *Edinburgh Evening Courant*, 28 October 1758.
8 *RPCS* v (1676–8), pp. 398–400.
9 J. Hajnal, 'European marriage patterns in perspective', in D.V. Glass and D.E.C. Everstey (eds.), *Population in History* (London, 1965), pp. 101–43; M.W. Flinn (ed.), *Scottish Population History from the Seventeenth Century to the 1930s* (Cambridge, 1977), pp. 271–83.
10 An Act of Parliament of 1649 added a parallel list of similar relationships created by marriage. This Act would have become invalid on the passing of the Act Rescissory of 1661, but it did not result in any change of the accepted rules, and part of the 1649 Act was re-stated in the Confession of Faith of 1690.
11 For the Confession of Faith, see *APS* ix 128, 133 and Appendix 147b.
12 Hugh Arnot, *A Collection and Abridgement of Celebrated Criminal Trials in Scotland*

from 1530 to 1784 (Edinburgh, 1785), pp. 307–11. Baron Hume states that the Tannahill decision was held by Lord Royston to be very doubtful, since it went beyond biblical wording and the bible was the basis of the definition of incest. David Hume, *Commentary on the Law of Scotland respecting Crimes* (Edinburgh, 1986), I, p. 446. The nullity decreet of 13 May 1825 – Kinninmount agt Rodger – is in the Commissary Court records, SRO.CC8/5/42 and CC8/6/144.

13 Hardy, 'The Attitudes of Church and State', Ch. 6; J.R. Cameron (ed.), *The First Book of Discipline* (Edinburgh, 1972), pp. 196–8.
14 This eventually led to the practice of not naming the paramour in the process of divorce, so that they could still marry. Hardy, 'The Attitudes of Church and State', Ch. 8; Patrick Fraser, *Treatise on the Law of Scotland as applicable to personal and domestic relations* (Edinburgh, 1846), I, pp. 686–9. But this did not happen until long after our period.
15 Hardy, 'The Attitudes of Church and State', Ch. 8; Sir George Mackenzie, *Law and Customs of Scotland in matters Criminal* (Edinburgh, 1678), p. 174.
16 J. Fergusson, *Treatise on the Present State of Consistorial Law in Scotland* (Edinburgh, 1829), Ch. 4.
17 For English parallels, see John R. Gillis, *For Better, For Worse: British Marriages, 1600 to the Present* (Oxford, 1985), pp. 52–4. In spite of its title this work does not cover Scotland.

4

Irregular Marriage

Besides regular marriage, which involved three public proclamations and a ceremony in the parish church, there was also irregular marriage. The irregularity lay solely in the way the union had been initiated, not in its legal status once established. The couple still had to be capable of marriage to each other (i.e. of age, not married to someone else, not within the forbidden degrees, and so on), and to have mutually consented to do so. An irregular marriage, once established, was as valid as any regular marriage; neither ecclesiastical nor civil law recognised an irregular *state* of marriage.

Both Church and State accepted marriages by what a lawyer would call *verba de praesenti,* that is the statement of consent by both parties, but proof was required. Witnesses would suffice, or letters from a man to a woman in which she was referred to as his wife. If a woman was customarily referred to as a man's wife in his presence and without contradiction, that was suggestive but not in itself enough to prove marriage.[1]

A further form of marriage accepted by the civil law was *verba de futuro,* a promise of marriage in the future, followed by sexual intercourse. Here again, proof of the promise would be required. Our cases suggest strongly that this form of marriage was not accepted by the Church. There were two cases in 1759, one in Troqueer, the other in Kilbrandon, where there clearly had been such a promise followed by intercourse, but the session accepted neither as marriages. In Troqueer the session exhorted the man 'to fulfil his Intentions of Marriage'; in Kilbrandon the session stopped the man marrying another woman and advised the girl to whom the promises had been made that she might pursue the man at law. If a couple wished such a marriage to be recognised by the Church all they had to do was declare their contract in public, which would make it a marriage *verba de praesenti.*

It has been alleged that there was a third form of irregular marriage in Scotland, 'by habit and repute'. Lawyers have considered this not as a separate form of marriage, but as a category of evidence by which marriage might be established. A couple living together and regarded as married could claim to be married by habit and repute, and the lawyers would say that at some time a promise would have been exchanged. It was very rarely that a claim for acceptance of such a marriage came up in church material; a couple who cohabited for any length of time could expect enquiry by the local session as to their marital status. Normally the couple would be asked to produce a certificate of marriage or a 'testificat' stating marriage from another parish. Correspondence would be initiated to enquire into the couple's background. However, in Dumfries (August 1696),

> James Allan, being brought before the session, with Janet Vetch whom he owned as his wife these eight years since they came from Ireland; And both of them

judicially acknowledged that they were never married, tho they have cohabited together as married persons these foresaid eight years, and have four children, and were reputed married persons in the place where they lived in Ireland before they came hither. Whereupon the session committed them to the Magistrate to be secured in prison untill they gave Baill to amend and satisfie for their continued fornication.

Had this happened in the eighteenth century they would certainly have been considered irregularly married.

In Longside (December 1749) Alexander Miller, now resident in Forfar, brought himself before the session with an unusual request. When he came over from France to fight in the 1745 rebellion he had met a woman, Helen Jordan, with whom he had cohabited in Longside parish, and she had borne a child to him, but he said that they had never married. He claimed that his reason for telling them this was in order to satisfy discipline for their fornication, after which he would marry her. The woman insisted they were married, and suspicion arose that Miller was trying to prove he had never been married to her so that he could marry another woman in Forfar. The session decided that:

Miller cannot be looked on as a free man but that he and said Helen Jordan are to be held married persons in regard they had of so long time been habit and repute such in this corner and had their child baptised upon the bona fide of said presumption – therefore they did and hereby do dismiss this process as invidious and unnatural on the man's part and as a design projected by him for obtaining marriage with another woman.

In Dalkeith (April 1770) Donald McDonald had been irregularly married to Helen Mckenzie; the session believed he was already married to another woman. The man declared he had cohabited with a woman called Christian Sword in the spring of 1769, 'and that his neighbours considered them as man and wife'. They had gone their separate ways during harvest, then cohabited for a further three weeks. She then went back to her parents in East Lothian, where he heard she had had a child, but he had had no further correspondence with her since then. The session decided that McDonald's cohabiting with Christian Sword 'amounted to a real Marriage' and forbade him to cohabit with Helen Mckenzie. The case was referred to presbytery, which concurred, and condemned his cohabitation with Helen Mckenzie as 'notour Adultery'.

According to folklore, there was another highly irregular type of marriage, 'handfasting'. This was said to be a system of temporary marriage, for up to a year and a day, which could be dissolved on the decision of the parties. All references to handfasting (even in the seventeenth century) place it in some vague and distant era,[2] and the myth probably arose from the practice of joining the hands of a couple at a public betrothal ceremony.[3]

In the cases above the existence of a marriage was inferred by the Church from the circumstance and behaviour of the couple. But in most cases the parties exchanged promises in front of a celebrant and witnesses, and were given some kind of marriage certificate. What made the marriage irregular was that the celebrant was not the parish minister of either participant, in fact often not a minister or priest at all, and there were no proclamations. Such a marriage could be 'bought' on a trip to town, avoiding the delay of proclamations, with no opportunity for either family to

4: Irregular Marriage

give its opinion on the match and without the local publicity which was a safeguard against bigamy. The motives for irregular marriage are discussed below: in short, there were some opportunists but most reflected a mixture of independence, convenience and fashion.

Irregular marriage carried statutory penalties. An Act of 1661 (consolidating Acts of the 1640s) ruled that the celebrator should be banished and those marrying were to be fined on a scale which ranged from 1,000 pounds Scots for a nobleman to 100 merks for a person of low status. The couple were liable also to three months in prison. A further Act of 1672 laid down that no one marrying to gain a dowry or an inheritance should receive them. This legislation may have been aimed at dissenters from the established Church rather than at the control of marriage, but in 1695 and 1698 the penalties were increased even though the laws against nonconformity had been repealed.[4] The statutes seem to have been attempts by the propertied classes to prevent their sons and heirs marrying against their wishes. In practice kirk sessions registered irregular marriage whenever it was reported and took a small fine from the couple. Whatever the law might say, it was undesirable to exact higher penalties for marriage than for fornication.

Legislation against irregular marriage thus bridged the change from an established episcopal Church to a presbyterian one in 1690. Those who wished to have the services of episcopalian clergy were forced into marrying irregularly. The position of some of these clerics became easier after the Toleration Act of 1712, which allowed them to conduct services provided they took the oaths of allegiance and prayed for the intruded royal family. But many of them remained Jacobite, and non-juring, and so liable to prosecution. In the absence of systematic work on sheriff court material, we cannot say how often episcopalian clergy were prosecuted, but there was one conspicuous case in 1755 when John Connachar was arrested in the Highlands for officiating as a minister and conducting a marriage without having taken the oaths. In spite of a defence which pointed out that there had been no qualified minister available within twenty miles, he was banished.[5] It is unlikely that any non-juring episcopalian minister would have been in trouble in the Highlands before 1746, provided he kept out of areas where the dominant clans were of Whig sympathies, but in the 1750s the government was nervous of any signs of Jacobitism in the Highlands, so the case reflects the political fears of the establishment rather than its views on irregular marriage.

In the seventeenth century marriages between Scots in England or in Ireland were also deemed irregular. After 1690 some couples might have been seeking an episcopal minister; others probably just wanted to escape the controls of the approved system. The Church's priority in our period was to have it clearly established whether a marriage had taken place: punishing those who had broken rules over the form or place of marriage took second place.

Though there are several seventeenth century instances of irregular marriage among the landed families of the Borders,[6] irregular marriage was otherwise almost non-existent before 1690, as Table 4.1 shows.

The figures in Table 4.1 are the numbers of irregular marriages registered by couples after the event, in those 78 parishes which we used for quantitative work. The base population for each regional sample will be 3,500 or more, for example the Border sample population was 5,000.[7]

Table 4.1 should not be used for comparisons between regions because of the

55

Table 4.1: Irregular marriages registered after the event
(from Webster's Census of 1755)

	Lothians	Fife	Central Lowlands	Central & Eastern Highlands	Western Highlands	Aberdeen-shire	North-east	Caithness	Ayrshire	South-west	Borders
Total population	3,492	7,277	8,191	10,334	6,724	7,954	8,269	3,780	4,517	4,101	4,968
1661–71	1	0	1	0	-	0	1	-	0	-	-
1671–80	0	0	4	0	0	0	0	0	0	8	-
1681–90	2	0	0	0	0	0	0	0	0	6	-
1691–1700	14	4	4	-	1	0	0	0	5	10	-
1701–10	15	9	8	-	1	1	3	0	3	19	-
1711–20	8	14	13	0	2	0	1	1	4	32	24
1721–30	48	18	20	0	2	1	1	1	5	30	40
1731–40	113	19	17	1	6	2	1	0	9	11	41
1741–50	78	21	16	2	6	2	3	0	1	25	48
1751–60	40	30	21	5	2	2	1	0	6	37	-
1761–70	83	67	25	1	15	2	0	0	4	49	77
1771–80	9	51	21	4	16	0	0	0	3	75	55

disparities between base populations, but it does show when irregular marriage became common in each region. In general, it was common in the south and rare in the north, though Ayrshire is an exception in being fairly low, and the West Highlands figure suddenly rises in the 1760s. There was a small increase in numbers of irregular marriages when the presbyterian establishment replaced the episcopal. In some instances this was doubtless due to principle; the refusal to be married by a presbyterian minister because of adherence to the Episcopal Church.[8] However, the more potent reason for the increase was the availability of deposed episcopal ministers who were willing to perform the marriage ceremony with few questions asked. The exceptional pattern of irregular marriage is that of the south-west, where proximity to the English border made it easy to slip across and get married by a Church of England minister.[9]

The real growth in irregular marriages began in the 1720s and accelerated from the 1730s. However, this only occurred in certain regions, and there is no obvious reason why irregular marriage sellers, as one might term them, might practise in certain areas but not in others. By the 1730s Edinburgh was the great irregular marriage centre of Scotland, and most couples residing in the Lothians, Fife and the Central Lowlands went to Edinburgh for their irregular marriages. The parishioners of South Leith, who were particularly prone to marry irregularly, also tended to do so in Edinburgh,[10] and even for couples in the eastern Highlands, Edinburgh was the place to go.

A port like Dundee seemed a logical place for irregular marriages to be conducted, so we examined the session records from the 1680s to 1750. Irregular marriage figures rose rapidly in the 1730s, and even more so in the 1740s, but virtually all those couples travelled to Edinburgh. Aberdeen had no irregular marriages to speak of, and Ayr parishioners travelled to Glasgow. The latter town was a minor centre for irregular marriages, and most West Highlanders seeking irregular marriage went there, or to Greenock.

Before the 1740s most of the irregular marriages in the south-west took place across the border in England, with the occasional one in Ireland or elsewhere in Scotland. However, from the 1740s onward Dumfries itself became a centre for irregular marriages, which spared couples the trek to England. As explained in the introduction, but it seemed worth looking at the irregular marriage traffic in the eastern borders. Before the 1730s, virtually all of the irregular marriages of Border couples were conducted by vicars in England. In the 1730s and 1740s most were still performed in England, but a growing number of couples went to Edinburgh instead; from the 1750s onward most of the certificates were signed at Edinburgh.

Absolute numbers indicate trends but not the proportion of total marriages which were irregular. Counting regular marriages in OPRs is very time-consuming and, given the state of many Scottish parish registers, is often not feasible, but we did look at a sub-sample of parishes where numbers of irregular marriages seemed high. The percentages are shown in Table 4.2.

In South Leith in the 1730s and 1740s, the irregular marriages even outnumbered the regular ones.[11]

In England irregular marriage came to a stop after Lord Hardwicke's Marriage Act, in March 1754. Thereafter, disobedient clery faced transportation for a first offence and death for repeat offences, and this effectively confined marriage in England to 'regular' procedures, which included the obtaining of parental consent for

Girls in Trouble

Table 4.2: Irregular marriages as percentage of total marriages

	Dysart (Fife)	Dalkeith (Lothians)	Cramond (Lothians)	Muiravonside (Central)	Troqueer (South-west)
1721–30	3.9	10.0			
1731–40	4.9	19.9	23.7		
1741–50	3.1	13.8	24.0	6.4	
1751–60	6.5		18.3	7.3	26.5
1761–70	13.2	29.2		10.3	25.9
1771–80	11.1			6.9	30.4

those under 21. A similar bill for Scotland was read once on 1 April 1755 but was then dropped, perhaps because of the opposition to the English Act.[12]

The resulting difference in marriage laws between the two countries created a pattern of runaway matches. Acquisitive men and wealthy heiresses from England could flee to the border, often pursued by indignant parents, and be married as soon as they were on Scottish soil, usually by a local innkeeper, who also benefited by other aspects of their custom. The favourite place for this was Gretna, but such matches also took place at other main road crossings, such as Coldstream Bridge and Lamberton Toll.[13]

Perhaps the publicity given to these English couples encouraged still more Scots to marry irregularly. Certainly by the 1760s irregular marriage, as Table 4.1 showed, was common in most regions.

The irregular celebration of marriage was made possible by the existence of individuals willing to perform such marriages. In the seventeenth century the only name which recurs (in Dumfries parish) is that of Christopher Knight, across the English border. In the early eighteenth century, however, when there was less risk of penalty, there were several deposed episcopal ministers who performed such marriages in Scotland. The two who appear to have done so most frequently in Edinburgh were Samuel Mowat and John Barclay.

Samuel Mowat first appears in the records in 1701 as 'late Episcopal Minister at Crawfordjohn' (elsewhere he is described as 'sometime Curat in Crawfordjohn'). His signature continues to appear on marriage certificates until as late as 1716, though he cannot have been as notorious as some other celebrators, for even at that date Wemyss session had doubts about a marriage testificat because 'they knew not if the said Samuel Muat be a Minister or not'.

A name which can be found more often is that of John Barclay, 'late Episcopal minister at Cockburnspath', who operated in the Canongate. The first mention of his name was in 1704 and the last in September 1711, when Cramond kirk session was warned by Edinburgh presbytery that Barclay

> does in ane Irregular and clandestin manner marry persons sometimes within the forbidden degrees, as also married men who had their wives alive at the time, and many are married by him without knowledge or consent of their parents, or proclamation of Bannes, as also that he gives false testimonialls, to cover the sin of uncleannesse, and being often cited to compeir and answer for the same, still refused, and never compeired.

Many of the points raised in this denunciation of Barclay will be discussed later in this chapter, but the point worth noting here is the inability of the presbytery to stop him.

Further west, the most notorious person in this period was Gilbert Mushet, deposed episcopal minister of Cumbernauld, who was allegedly deposed 'for swearing cursing fighting, drinking and many Irregular marriages of unfree persons'.[14] He normally operated in Cumbernauld (though at least one Rothesay couple were married by him at Largs); and couples from as far afield as Torphichen in West Lothian, Muthill in Lowland Perthshire, St Ninians in Stirling, and Ayr town, were married by him, from the beginning of the eighteenth century until about 1716. Muthill session recorded an irregular marriage in 1712 by Mushet, 'alias cuple the beggars'.

In the south-west from 1711 onwards some couples were married by a Mr Hugh Clanny, but Dumfries session recorded that in March 1717 he was jailed for this, awaiting prosecution before the next Circuit Court. In the eastern borders, Kelso session recorded in November 1713 that one James Miller, minister at Lowick in Northumberland, frequently came to Kelso 'and marries severall persons most unwarrantablie & disorderly, which may prove of fatal consequence by encouraging many young women to disobey their parents, & altogether contemn their authority, by marrying to dragoons, & other idle persons, whereby they expose themselves to great misery to the grief & heavy affliction of their parents'; the town baillie was to apprehend the man and imprison him if he was found 'about such business'. Miller continued celebrating irregular marriages through the 1720s but did so on his own side of the border. In the 1730s two well-established and conveniently placed English vicars – Thomas Ogle at Carham and Thomas Drake at Norham – performed almost all the over-the-border marriages.

Apart from the rogue ministers, there were even sleazier individuals who 'performed marriages'. In St Ninians (June 1723), Alexander Cleveland said he had been married by 'a Nottar who dwelt at the tron at the south end of the toun' called Mackie. According to Cleveland, Mackie had gone off 'to sollicit the Curat to do it' and when he returned told him

> that the Curat would not do it under a guiney and added moreover that he would do it much cheaper for he had done it to severals formerly whereupon the said Alexander returning with Mackie was married by him in his house at the Tron and another partie from Dunblane one after ane other that they might be witnesses to each other who haveing used a forme of prayer spoke of the duties and made them join hands and then declared them married persons and ther they stayed all night till each partie drank about a crown and then he did give them a testificat of their marriage in name of some other as if he had not done it.

In the 1730s no one matched the industry of David Strange (or Strang), who carved out something of a monopoly trade in irregular marriage in Edinburgh, and hence for most of Scotland. In 1739 Dysart session refused to baptise the child of a couple married by Strange without a sponsor 'in regard that Mr Strang is under the sentence of excommunication'. In 1738 Cramond session rebuked a couple who had been married by him 'for having recourse to an Infamous person for Marriage', and another pair in 1739 for 'being married by an abandoned & excommunicated person'. Cramond session also recorded in September of that year that Strange had

Girls in Trouble

been banished from Scotland, and his name disappears from the records for a year or two. (As is related in *Sin in the City,* further research revealed that he was simply using an alias during that period.) In 1742 he was again trading under his own name, but by that time he had competition from a number of other 'marriage sellers'.

Certain names recur throughout the 1740s, 1750s, and 1760s: John Grierson, George Blaikie, William Jamieson, Patrick Douglas, and David Paterson. In 1743 Pencaitland session sharply rebuked a couple married by Paterson 'for being thus irregularly married by a person who never had been a Minister & who was justly Excommunicate for pretending to be one and acting as one & for other wicked & scandalous practices'. Irregular marriers in Leith in the 1770s and 1780s have been traced via Edinburgh directories, and can be seen to have had other sources of income. John Stewart was a sheriff substitute, Thomas Murray and Charles Johnston were schoolmasters.[15]

At least such men – and their signatures – were known to the Church, which helped to distinguish the irregular but valid marriages from the forgeries and frauds. In Forgandenny in March 1742, James Rintoul and Janet Marshal produced marriage lines signed by David Williamson at Edinburgh. The session thought that the lines were forged 'because of some very great Informalities in them and also because never any of them had ever heard of one under forsaid Name in or about Edinburgh that used to mary People in the Clandestine Way'; they refused to accept the marriage without further proof. At the end of May the minister reported that when he was in Edinburgh for the General Assembly,

> he was very certainly informed by Persons he could credit that there was a Man in or about Edinburgh that made a Practice of marrying People in a Clandestine way and subscribed the Marriage Lines he gave them David Williamson Minr tho' 'twas generally believed that was not his true name but that for his Security and the more Secrecy he had changed his name.

After additional attestations by reliable churchmen, the marriage was accepted. ('Williamson' was, in fact, David Strange, who disguised his signature too well.)

This degree of tolerance of irregular marriers may seem surprising, but less so in view of what occurred in Muthill parish in 1743. Two couples had been irregularly married 'by one Douglas who never was Minister of any Denomination'. The session 'resolved to apply to som proper judges to cause that Douglas to be apprehended and punished according to Law'. Douglas was indeed apprehended, only to be freed by the judge in Crieff who refused to take the matter any further. As early as 1701, Dumfries session fulminated:

> albeit Civil Magistrates of the Bounds have been frequently addressed, & have sometimes promised to take Course with such persons Irregularly Married, Yet they have hitherto neglected to Execute the Laws against them; Yea some of these Magistrates, Instead of punishing, have by sham-fineing in some small fine (which was either never Exacted, or not bestowed as apointed by Law) endeavoured to protect the Delinquents.

If the civil authorities were refusing to back up church courts in prosecuting such men, then the Church just had to learn to live with them.

By the 1760s the lucrative practice was even corrupting the established Church. Kelso session recorded with horror instances of an Edinburgh session clerk or depute clerk, bribed to sign a testificat stating that a couple were resident in the parish and had been duly proclaimed – even when the couple themselves never claimed such a thing – so that the parish minister would, in ignorance, marry them in his church.[16]

How did kirk sessions resolve the more dubious claims of marriage? Suppose, for example, a woman produced a testificat of an irregular marriage to a soldier who had already left the parish. If it was a straightforward document, properly witnessed and signed, then the woman was usually accepted as married. But a pregnant woman whose soldier partner had gone off with his regiment might well make a false claim. In Kingsbarns in 1710 Janet Philp, craving baptism for her child, said she had been married to the father, Thomas Alexander, a soldier, when he was stationed at Leith. The minister refused baptism 'because of the insufficiency of her testificat'. The session, joined for the inquiry by two ministers from the presbytery, found

> several contradictions betwixt Janet Philps confession and the alledged testificat of her marriage, first, as to the date of her marriage, secondly as to the womans name she being called in the testificat Jean Philp whereas she calls herself Jannet Philp, thirdly as to the name of the Minister she calling him Mr Barklay and the testificat John Bartholomew besides other informalities in the testificat.

The woman eventually confessed she was not married but guilty of fornication. When asked 'how she had come to that forged testificate of marriage she answered it was sent to her enclosed in a letter from some of Thomas Alexanders Comerads whose name(s) she knew not'. Dundee saw two cases in 1748 and 1749 of women producing 'marriage certificates' which were forged by soldiers; it was by no means an uncommon occurrence.

In the period when irregular marriages were uncommon sessions took a very cautious line, demanding watertight certificates or witnesses to the marriage. When neither acceptable certificates nor witnesses were forthcoming sessions usually referred to the presbytery for advice, and the presbytery would say that if the couple swore publicly to adhere to one another the marriage should be accepted. Examples could be produced from almost any part of the country, the earliest occurring in Cramond in 1698.

By the mid-eighteenth century most kirk sessions were taking the same line as presbyteries, that it was the couple's public declaration of adherence rather than the ceremony or documentation that mattered. Two examples will suffice. When a couple appeared in Eskdalemuir parish in 1737, the session, deciding that their testimonial 'could not be depended on, it looking like a forged one the names of the Witnesses & pretended Celebrator appearing all to be writ by the same hand &c agreed that they should be rebuked publickly and declare their adherence to each other as husband & wife'. In Muthill in 1768 a couple 'produc'd some confus'd Lines of Marriage altogether unintelligible – In presence of the Session they testified their mutual Willingness and Inclination as Man & Wife – The Minister exhorted and rebuk'd them, declared them married persons and dismiss'd them.'

The ease with which sessions were accepting irregular marriages by this time is clear from two cases in Troqueer parish. In the first, in 1753, a couple 'confessed that they were Irregullarly Maried. But produced no testimony thereof but their own assertion'. This marriage was accepted, as was that of 1760 when a couple confessed 'they were Irregularly Married Eight days ago, in the open fields near Bridgend of Dumfries, by one whom they did not know, & whose name they did not ask That

Girls in Trouble

they gave him a Guinea for Marrying them.'

However, if both parties were not present and willing to make such a declaration, the session had to rely on other evidence, such as a letter in which the man acknowledged the woman as his wife. In Inveraray (June 1748) Mary Walker came to the session, seeking baptism for her child. She said she was married to the father, an Irishman and a soldier, and produced two letters from him. The session was at first hesitant, 'not knowing whither they were genuine', but after she made further appearances, including one before presbytery, it accepted her as married.

In a case in Banff (December 1758) Isabel Murray claimed she was married to David Frigge, merchant, but that he refused to acknowledge her as his wife. Frigge had forced her to sign a paper renouncing her claim to him as her husband, but she still held a series of letters signed 'Your Affectionate Husband'. The case was referred to presbytery, which ruled that:

> as the Law of the Land with respect to Marriage is extremely plain, and as it as plainly appears to us, that there is a full and explicit consent of marriage and marriage plainly implied between the said Parties in the Letters laid before us, and as the said David Frigge did not refuse these Letters before the Kirk Session of Banff, and has not chosen to attend the Presbytery to advance any thing against the authority and effect of these letters, the Presbytery judged that they had all Reason to hold the Letters as good and to have been really wrote and signed by the said David Frigge, They therefore thought themselves fully warranted to assoilzie... the said Isabel Murray from the Scandal of Fornication as laid in the Reference. But at the same time from the Confession of the said Isabel Murray, and as none of the Parties adduce any Proof of a regular Marriage, they find their Marriage must have been clandestine, for which they are as yet censurable.

The other category of evidence, rarely used, was that of 'habit and repute', i.e. that because of their behaviour to each other everyone acquainted with a particular couple believed them to be married, whether or not there was written proof. In Lochgoilhead (November 1752) Colin McEwen and Catharine McKellar declared they were irregularly married in Glasgow and produced lines. 'The lines did not appear at all likely or sufficient but as they had Cohabite so long together and Publickly acknowledged themselves Married Persons the Session Determined to look on them henceforward as Such.' A similar judgment was made in Spott in 1767, and in Dalkeith (December 1769) the actual wording was used. Margaret Innis, seeking her child's baptism, said she had been irregularly married to John Scott but that he had left her. Apart from a certificate, she was able to produce neighbours who declared 'That they knew that they lived in the same house and were in habit and repute in the Neighbourhood to be man and wife.'

In Dysart (April 1780) Charles Arrot, a soldier, asked for baptism 'for his child brought forth by Elizabeth Patoun whom he calls his wife'. The minister informed the session that Arrot's officer

> had signified by a Line that he had lived with the said woman as his wife since June last – The man owned he had not been married because his officer would not give him a Line because he did not desire the men to have wives, – and that without such line none would proclaim him – He was rebuked for the irregularity of his marriage & allowed Baptism for his Child.

4: Irregular Marriage

The phraseology of this case is interesting because it is clear that no marriage ceremony of any kind took place, and the session was therefore considering habit and repute alone to make an irregular marriage.

'Habit and repute' were particularly invoked in Kelso in the 1770s. In July 1771 George Wood and Christian Bold produced a certificate of their marriage dated at Edinburgh in April of that year,

> tho' by their own acknowledgement they received it at Coldstream, so stupidly written that no regard could be paid to it. But as it was known to the members of the Session, and inhabitants of this place, that they have lived as married persons since that Date they were rebuked for their irregularity severely, and exhorted as Christians to live in the married State.

The certificate of John Fox and Margaret Turnbull, dated 6 February 1744, was 'so strangely written that no regard could be paid to it; but it having been known & attested that they had lived in this place habit & repute as man & wife since about the beginning of Febr last' the marriage was accepted. Many more examples could be produced, and by the end of the decade cohabitation was the standard test of irregular marriage in Kelso. It was, however, the only session of those we looked at which took this line. By contrast, in Troqueer, in the south-west, as late as the 1760s and 1770s more than one couple appearing before the session insisted they had not yet cohabited 'because they wanted to satisfy the session for their Irregular Marriage previous to any Cohabitation'.

Why did the kirk sessions spend so much time on irregular marriages? One reason was the Church's wish to maintain its authority, which was becoming eroded as the eighteenth century wore on. The social norm of being married solely in the parish kirk after the proclamation of banns was being undermined; by summoning irregularly married couples sessions asserted a measure of control. Baptism was the Church's strongest lever, for baptism continued to be very important to parents, and their child would not be baptised until they were in good standing with the session.[17] However, the Church's concern was not merely self-serving; it also tried to protect the innocent. There were no doubts about the status of a couple who had been proclaimed and married in church, but any other kind of alleged marriage could involve frivolity or deception.

In Stranraer (March 1774) Janet Campbell declared she had been married a fortnight earlier to John Mean, skipper of the Pelikan Sloop, in the house of Alexander McWhinnie, ships carpenter, and that they had lain together as man and wife. She further declared that on a subsequent date, in the presence of witnesses, he had asked her to deny the marriage, which she refused to do. Mean compeared and admitted being in McWhinnie's house that night, but said he had been so drunk he remembered nothing of what had happened. He had

> since been told that Janet Campbell came into the Company while he was there, upon which as he imagines his Commerades wanting to divert themselves with him carried him upstairs and threw him into a Bed along with the said Janet Campbell; but that he knew not whether she is Man, or Woman, for he had no Commerce with her as a Woman and that he knows Nothing of a Marriage and that he had no Intention to be married that Day to any Woman, much less to her whom he had never seen before.

Girls in Trouble

As for the subsequent meeting, he declared 'he had no such conversation with her as she alledges, only he offered her a Dram if she would tell him who helped to carry off his two Barrels of Herrings she had taken from the Shore.' Finally he declared he was very sorry 'for having been drunk, and for any Indecencies he may have been guilty of in Consequence of his Drunkenness'. He convinced the session that there had been no marriage, and that his later conversation was solely about the herring.

In Kinglassie (April 1759), Helen Smith showed the session a certificate of marriage to John Lauchlan, but it was put to her that she was supposedly already married: in 1753 she had gone off with a soldier, George Murray, and when she returned she had told the session she had been irregularly married to a Robert Roberts, though she had never produced any evidence. Her story now was that 'a certain Friend of hers had feign'd the whole story of a marriage with Robert Roberts and had prevailed with her to narrate it to the Session for fear of Censure upon the report of her having gone away to Leeth in company with George Murray... & she pled that she was then so young as to be easily prevaild with to tell any Thing to save her from the Censure of the Kirk'. The session accepted her story,

> that from the mere fear of Censure she had been imposed on to narrate of the story of a marriage with Roberts & that it was entirely groundless and they agreed she should be rebuked for her indecency in following George Murray, her falsehood in narrating the story of her marriage with Roberts & her irregularity in her clandestine marriage with Lauchlan.

In the above cases the ambiguities of irregular marriage did not have any lasting consequences, but often a man tried to repudiate an irregular marriage. In Troqueer (July 1748) Margaret Reid admitted there had been no witnesses to her marriage with Robert Rogerson, but she had marriage lines and had cohabited with him. Rogerson 'absolutely denied that ever he was Married regularly or Irregularly to the said Margaret Reid he likeways Refused that he had ever cohabited with hir and that what she had said about the Marriage lines was altogether false & groundless'. The woman in whose house they had spent their wedding night testified that she had been unwilling to allow them to share a bed until Rogerson had declared he had married Margaret Reid that same evening. He continued to deny the marriage in spite of other witnesses' declarations that he had slept in one bed with her and referred to her as his wife. In January 1750 he was publicly rebuked 'for his gross prevarication Dissimulation and Equivocation upon oath'. The session certainly considered them married, but it is not clear if it ever got the man to acknowledge the woman as his wife.

In St Ninians (September 1726) James Gibson, who some years earlier had produced a certificate of his irregular marriage with Isobell Hendry, and later presented their children for baptism, now insisted that the certificate had been forged and he had never been married to her. The woman affirmed they had been married, and the case was referred to presbytery which 'sustained them as married persons'. In two of the other cases we found of a man attempting to repudiate the woman he had married irregularly (Troqueer, March 1753 and April 1776) there was a further complication in the shape of another woman whom the man now claimed as his wife.

Amongst the motives for marrying irregularly, deception and bigamy (what we might term serial monogamy) looms very large. A typical case is that of Mary Black (Troqueer, September 1767), who confessed she had been irregularly married to William Pitchfurth, a soldier, and that she did cohabit with him as his wife for some time, but that afterwards he destroyed their Marriage-lines & left her. And... sometime after they were married that she heard some of his fellow-soldiers say, that he had a wife in England, tho the said William denyed to her that he was married to any other woman.

Those fellow soldiers confirmed to the session that Pitchfurth had a wife in England, so Mary Black was not held to be a married woman.

In a similar case (Kilmartin January 1761), Christian Smith had been irregularly married to Duncan McUrachadair, a soldier, who 'was married to another woman who was in life at the time of his marriage with her'. She was asked

> how she came to marry a man whom for ought she knew might be married to another woman, answer'd that she was imposed upon for that he produced a Letter testifying that his former wife died sometime before and was decently interr'd and hoped this would alleviate her fault. The session taking the Premises under their Consideration they found her too credulous and rash in a matter of such weight yet made some allowance for her being impos'd upon.

However, it treated her as an adulteress.

The brevity of yet another such tale does not disguise its sadness. In Dalkeith (November 1742), Janet Mortoun acknowledged she had been irregularly married to Arthur Wier, 'and that she went with her Child to him at Glasgow, and stayed, untill such time as another woman to whom he was married in Ireland, came to him, and they both went off together to Ireland, and she and her child were left to return home.'

An equally sad case revealing how women, with their low literacy rates, could be exploited was that of Katharine Sooty in Wemyss (January 1737). She returned from harvest stating that she had been married to James Ogilvie, a soldier, 'who made her believe his wife he had last was dead, and he a widower, that she had cohabit with him as his lawful wife, till his wife, who he said was dead, came seeking him, which made him flee and leave them both.' When asked, 'If she had any marriage lines to show? Yes replyed she, and gave in a paper, which she said, she got from him, and which he called marriage lines: Which being read, it was a summonds he had got for a certain debt.'

But not all women were credulous innocents. In Wemyss (February 1759), Elspet Wemyss was caught in bed with John Taylor when the press gang burst in and carried him off. She said she was married to him, 'that at the time of their marriage she knew that he had other two wives then alive, & that she intended her marriage should have been kept secret till after the death of the other wife he has in this Country, had it not been accidentally discovered by a Letter of his to her being intercepted'. Although it was the man, not the woman, who had contracted three marriages, presbytery considered her guilty of polygamy, though she fled before discipline could be imposed.

In Troqueer (December 1763), James Thomson claimed that his former wife, Ann Crosbie, was dead and that he had been irregularly married nine months earlier to Jain Chalmers, with whom he cohabited. The session were informed 'that the relations of Ann Crosbie Declare that she was alive last summer and that they have never heard of hir death.' Here there was intentional fraud, but in other cases there was genuine doubt or mistake. In Moulin (August 1761), Donald Drummond and

Girls in Trouble

Girzel Cunison were clandestinely married, though Drummond had been married before. Some years earlier his wife

> became greatly Disordered in her Judgment, travelled, Distracted thro' the world; left this country [i.e. region] entirely, & has not been seen in it, for near five years past; but still there is no Evidence of her being Dead; & it is said, & believed in the Country, that she was seen in Life by Persons that knew her in Argyleshire within two years past.

In Muiravonside (July 1769), John Dick, who married Janet Cochran irregularly, declared his former wife had been 'a bad woman with other Men' and went off with a soldier eight years earlier. He had since 'heard by transient Report that she was dead and that he had caused call her at several Mercat Towns but could not hear any account of her and thereupon thought that he was in safety to Marry a second time.' In Kelso (May 1766), James Wilson married Elizabeth Hutchison irregularly. He had no proof of his first wife's death, but he 'had lived ten years in Kelso without hearing from her & that he left her on account of her lewd and wicked life – and had reason to believe she was dead.' In all three of the above cases the sessions involved did not uphold the second marriages, and the cases were all referred to the relevant presbyteries. Unfortunately we were not able to discover the outcomes.

Women did not often desert their husbands; it was usually men who vanished. Cases of women whose husbands had left them years earlier and who now wished to remarry occur throughout our period, and the woman was always required to produce evidence of her first husband's death before the second marriage would be accepted. The earliest we found was in Dysart in 1669 (March–August), where George Dole and Isoball Weems had married irregularly in England. There was doubt about her former husband's death, and the case went as far as synod, but synod could only advise, as presbytery had done, that they be prohibited to cohabit until the evidence was forthcoming. Eventually, at the woman's request, the minister wrote to the captain of the company in which her former husband, Andrew Tyrie, had been a soldier, and learned

> that Andrew Tyrie was indeed one of the souldiours of his company and that having killed his neighbour he had fled and after that tyme he never heard more of him The Session judge that ther is a probability he is alive because it wold appear the only barre that keeps him from returning is the conviction he hes of murther and the fear of his lyfe therfor.

George Dole and Isoball Weems were treated as adulterers.

In Ayr (August 1692), Nance Cunningham, when asked how she could remarry when it was reported her 'latter husband' was still alive, was emphatic that 'she knew very well that he was dead, because she had spoken with severall persons who had come from that Isle where he died and was at his buriall.' Proving the death of a husband who had disappeared was difficult and, as noted in the last chapter, divorce for desertion was not attempted by any woman in a rural parish in our period.

The incentive this gave to marry irregularly was well expressed in a case in Banff (January 1705). Norman Denoon was asked how he could marry a woman

> of whose husband's death there was no legal document, to all which the said Norman made answer, that he had made all possible search for a Testificate of her

first husband's death & went to Edinburgh for that effect did (as it seems) gett some persons who did give some declaratione that way before an Episcopall incumbent there, who did marry the said Norman & Isabell, & being again interrogate why he did not proceed regularly in his marriage with an established Minister of the Government, made answer that he doubted they would accept so frankly of the declaration given anent the death of her Husband.

However, as an irregular marriage still had to be ratified by the kirk session, which would demand proof of a former spouse's death, a couple were likely to be separated and treated as adulterers unless they produced such proof.

Of the 27 cases we collected of bigamous irregular marriages, only eight took place before 1740, the remaining nineteen occurring between 1741 and 1780. This might be the result of increased opportunities for travel, and hence for desertion, but it might also indicate a greater inclination to ignore the traditional rules.

The Church feared not only bigamy but that a couple irregularly married might be within the prohibited degrees of kinship and affinity, in other words the relationship might be incestuous. However, we found only two such cases. The first occurred in Stranraer, in December 1744. The woman was her husband's 'grand niece from the same father but not from the same mother, but from a second marriage, so that her grand mother was his own half sister'. The case was referred to presbytery who declared this to be incest and forbade them to cohabit. In Muiravonside (July 1771), the woman concerned was 'full niece' to the man's former wife. Presbytery ordered them to separate, but the man declared, 'whom God had put together, no man should put asunder' and refused to do so. Eventually a sentence of lesser excommunication was pronounced on the couple.

Another motive for irregularly marrying was to get a certificate that predated pregnancy in order to avoid church discipline for 'antenuptial fornication'. In January 1779 the kirk session of Mauchline, inveighing against celebrators of irregular marriages, condemned the way 'such persons do frequently if not always impose on the publick, particularly the Church Judicatories by forging or antedating marriage Lines in Order to conceal Antinuptial fornication.'

Such antedated certificates do surface at various times, but in our period kirk sessions knew too much about their parishioners for this to work. In July 1716, in Kelso, John Lorrain and Marion Nisbet produced a testificat of marriage dated 3 May. The session was 'jealous that it is antedated and that they went away only yesterday to be married'; two months later the couple confessed this was so. In Wemyss, in February 1721, the minister refused to baptise the child of James Watson and Margaret Youel 'in regard he suspected the Testimonial of their marriage antedated'. The man declared he had been married on 3 April 1720. He was grilled by the minister about where he had lodged on his wedding night and why he did not own his marriage at that time, and replied, 'he knew no reason for that, seeing he was immediately going to sea, and had not a house and other things provided, his wife therefore went to service; and as soon as he came home in November last, he owned his marriage'. The session demanded witnesses to his marriage; he said he could not produce them because one was dead and the other out of town. Nothing daunted, the session told him to get an attestation from the minister at South Leith that there were reliable witnesses to marriage taking place on 3 April, otherwise the testimonial would not be accepted and they would be referred to the Justices of Peace. Two months later the woman confessed they had not married until 25 November and had been guilty of antenuptial fornication. This session was unusually assiduous in pursuit of the case, but kirk sessions did not like being taken for fools.

In another Fife case (Dysart 1722), William Stewart and Helen Cout clearly had failed to obtain an antedated marriage certificate. On 7 October the man craved baptism for a newborn child, saying he had been married a year ago 'but knew not who it was that married them and that the brieff of his marriage was lost'. The minister insisted he must prove his marriage or else be considered a fornicator. A month later the certificate was produced, dated 28 May, 'by which the session find them guilty of antenuptial fornication and lying and dissembling with the session'.

In Dundee in November 1733 John Simons and Margaret Brown produced a certificate signed by David Strange and dated 15 May. The session refused to accept such a document with the ink barely dry, and the couple confessed that in fact they had been married the previous Wednesday, 21 November. The session did not validate the marriage until months later when the couple produced another line signed by Strange, with the correct date on it. In Pencaitland in 1753, a couple cited on 28 October produced a marriage certificate dated 20 June but admitted they had married on 6 October. The session register records that it was 'pretty evident that Agnes Sanderson was far gone with child'. Concealment of antenuptial pregnancy, all the same, was not a frequent motive for irregular marriage. As shown in Chapter 5, levels of antenuptial pregnancy were generally low. The truth usually emerged in any case. More significantly, we found a large number of cases where couples admitted at the same time (or within a short space of time) both to irregular marriage and to antenuptial fornication, which they would not have done if their reason for marrying irregularly had been to conceal their prenuptial sexual activities.

Episcopal sentiments were mentioned earlier as a motive for irregular marriage, and there were other religious differences as well, particularly when the man (no such women were discovered) was Roman Catholic. We found Roman Catholic men marrying irregularly in the north-east, the south-west, the Lothians and the Central Lowlands. In Cramond (January 1732), John Clerk 'confest he was married by one of his own way of thinking, that he had no lines of Marriage because their Minister uses to give none, but that he could produce witnesses to their Marriage if need shou'd require it'. The session, 'considering this to be a singular case and how contrary to the Laws of this Kingdom for a popish priest to marrie persons', referred the case to presbytery. Presbytery advised the session to examine the witnesses and if satisfied to rebuke the couple for their irregular marriage. The couple could not produce the witnesses, so presbytery then recommended that if the couple adhered to their marriage the session should accept it.

Most irregular marriages with a Roman Catholic were celebrated not by a priest but by those Edinburgh 'ministers' or laymen who plied the irregular marriage trade. There may also have been a private religious ceremony, but it was the certificate supplied by the irregular minister which enabled the marriage to be accepted by the session. Indeed, it was the rules of the Church that frustrated regular marriages in such cases. In Muthil (July 1760) Margaret Key was rebuked 'for marrying a Papist', and the session clerk recorded that 'They had been refused Proclamation of Banns as is usual in such cases conform to act of Session.' In New Abbey (Jan 1770) Stewart McPherson, a Roman Catholic, had asked to be proclaimed for marriage with Agnes McKie, a Protestant; when the minister refused, they went off and married irregularly. In both cases, although the minister had refused to marry the couples

4: Irregular Marriage

regularly, the irregular marriage was accepted as valid.

An important motive for irregular marriage was parental opposition. As was noted in Chapter 3, although parental consent was not a legal requirement, parental pressure could be difficult to withstand. Parents had various means of influence: scolding and emotional blackmail, a refusal to help with material goods or a portion,[18] and in some cases a refusal to admit an errant child to share in a tenancy or craft position. The child might prefer to present them with a fait accompli than face a slow drip of opposition.

In a seventeenth-century case – long before irregular marriage became commonplace – we found that although the couple involved did not mention parental opposition, the session clearly considered that to be an important and understandable motive. This was in Dalkeith (October 1670), where Andrew Fleming and Janat Mitchelson were 'charged with the scandalous and unorderlie way which they had taken to accomplish theire marriage which they might have done with far more credit at home and lesse offence to the people of God Especially theire being no such disparitie between them or theire fortunes but they might have easilie procured the consent of all parties enterested'.

In two cases in the 1690s parental opposition was specifically mentioned. In Dysart (July 1695), when John Brown was asked why he had gone from the parish to marry Jean Gairdner 'seeing they might had the benefit of mariag hear answered that her parrents wold not allow her to marrie him'. In Dumfries (April 1698), John Irving and Agnes Duff were married 'beyond the border'; they acknowledged their fault, 'pretending withall, that they were forced to that course by her Mother who was against their marriage'. In Dumfries, in 1722, two of the couples who married irregularly not only did not have their parents' consent, but were also under age. After referral to presbytery both marriages were accepted as valid.

These situations continued through the eighteenth century. In Troqueer (September 1763) David Fergusson and Agnes Stott 'declared that the Reluctance of Agnes Stotts Mother & that of hir other friends to this Marriage was the Rasone why they married Irregularly'. Also in Troqueer (February 1764), James Ewing and Grizel Alexander added after their confession 'that they would have published their Irregular Marriage long ago had it not been that the said Grizels Relations were very averse to hir Marriage with the Said James Ewing.' A Dundee couple (March 1733), married by David Strange in Edinburgh, 'being Interrogate if they hade consent of Parents answered they hade not for hade they hade that they would not have troubled Mr Strange.'

Some couples may have wanted to escape the whole tedious business of a regular marriage, and from the drunken japes and customs, 'penny weddings' for instance, or the procession outside the church at East Linton described in 1725 where a cake was ritually broken over the head of the bride. We did not find any couples giving such a reason for marrying irregularly, but in Dunbarney (November 1698) the beadle complained 'that the Collections att Marriages being his due he sustains losse by severall persones, who tho they should be married in this place yet for privacie chose rather to goe in to the toun of Perth and therefore desireing that the Session would condescend upon for preventing his losse'.

A last minute change of mind would have made a 'private' marriage desirable. Two such cases surfaced in Kelso. In December 1728 James Ker irregularly married a woman who was betrothed to his own brother. In February 1740 Jean Ker married

Girls in Trouble

William Lockie in England, though she had been proclaimed twice with another man.

Some couples married irregularly because they were in a great hurry or for various other reasons. Ann Seaton and Peter Mckenzie appeared before Troqueer session (November 1764) to confess their irregular marriage, and explained that 'as the said Peter was obliged to go to Glasgow tomorrow to joyn the Regement there they had not time to be Regularly proclamed and Married.' Another Troqueer couple, Robert Stot and Isabell Carlyle (November 1764) 'said they would have Married Regularly had the said Robert not been obliged to sail to Whitehaven upon Monday or Tuesday night'. In an unusual Highland case (Kilmartin, November 1734), Donald Campbell of Barmaddy abducted Margaret Campbell, daughter of Dugald Campbell of Kilmartin, and took her to the Lowlands where they were clandestinely married. He admitted 'that he carried away the Forementioned Margaret Campbell, sore against her will though afterwards he obtained her consent'. In Rothesay in 1772 Mary McDonald married Samuel Saunders, 'a negroe man late the property of Mr Campbell'.

There were couples with pressing reasons, couples with shady reasons, and, perhaps more typical, couples with no particular reason at all. David McKie and Agnes Hannay (Wigtown, December 1722) 'could give no rational account why they married irregularly after two proclamations in this Church'. It should be emphasised that sessions seldom tried to ascertain the reason for a couple's marrying irregularly; their concern was whether a marriage existed. That said, we believe there was simply a fashion for irregular marriage, especially as many of these couples could just as easily – perhaps even more easily – have got married in their own parish church. If one's friends and acquaintances were getting married in this way, then perhaps one followed suit. Like all fashions, it passed, and the figures for irregular marriages did not continue to rise during the nineteenth century. But irregular marriage emerges as one of the main reasons for the breakdown of discipline in the late eighteenth century. If legally married couples could live together without declaring their status to the Church, it became harder for sessions to act against those producing illegitimate children.

Secular tolerance of irregular marriage sellers aided the trade and, by not following the English strictures of Harwicke's Marriage Act, the civil law was an indirect cause of loss of Church authority. Further observations on the relationship between the secular and ecclesiastical positions in our period must await research on Declarator of Marriage cases in the Commissary Court records.

Our cases show the extreme ease of marrying in Scotland. If two people without impediment stated in front of their kirk session that they married each other, then married they were. It is against this facility of marriage that illegitimacy has to be seen.

Notes

1 Ronald D. Ireland, 'Husband and Wife', in *Introduction to Scottish Legal History* (Stair Society, Edinburgh, 1958), pp. 82–9; J.R. Hardy, 'The Attitudes of Church and State in Scotland to Sex and Marriage' (unpublished M.Phil. thesis, Edinburgh University, 1978). Failure to recognise that Church and State used different law is responsible for some confusion in Patrick Fraser, *Treatise on the Law of Scotland as applicable to Personal and*

4: Irregular Marriage

Domestic Relations (Edinburgh, 1846), I, p. 334 on irregular marriage.
2   Martin Martin, *Description of the Western Isles of Scotland* (Glasgow, 1884), p. 124; T. Pennant, *Tour in Scotland* (London, 1790), II, pp. 91–7.
3   A.E. Anton, 'Handfasting in Scotland', *Scottish Historical Review xxxvii* (1958), pp. 89–102; T.C. Smout, 'Scottish Marriage, Regular and Irregular, 1500–1940', in R.B. Outhwaite (ed.), *Marriage and Society* (London, 1981), p. 211.
4   *APS* v 348 (1641) viii 184 (1649) vii 231(1661) viii 71B (1672) ix 387 (1695) and x 149B (1698). The 1695 and 1698 statutes imposed further tariffs of fines on couples marrying irregularly, ranging from 2,000 pounds Scots to 200 merks. In 1698 a fine of 100 pounds was levied on witnesses, and the celebrator of marriage could suffer corporal or pecuniary punishment at the will of the Privy Council.
5   Hugh Arnot, *A Collection and Abridgement of Celebrated Criminal Trials in Scotland from AD 1536 to 1784* (Edinburgh, 1785). pp. 331–40; *Scots Magazine 1755,* pp. 307–9, 311–16.
6   K. and H. Kelsall, *Scottish Lifestyle 300 Years Ago* (Edinburgh, 1987).
7   The parishes used for the Borders region are Longformacus, Sprouston, Yetholm and Kelso.
8   It is curious that although Dumfries kirk session (the only parish in this region for which records exist for the 1670s and 1680s) cited the couples for irregular marriage, the marriages were not regarded as valid: each couple had to be proclaimed and married *de novo* before being allowed to cohabit. In all the records we examined this was the only parish and period with such an attitude and procedure.
9   In Dundee there were no irregular marriages in this period, but two acts were passed by the session (August 1700 and August 1702) attempting to stop the practice by which couples were legally proclaimed three times in the parish church and then went and got married by an episcopal minister.
10 James Scott Marshall, 'Irregular Marriages in Scotland as Reflected in Kirk Session Records', *Records of the Scottish Church History Society 18* (1972–4), pp. 10–25, and also (ed.), *Calendar of Irregular Marriages in the South Leith Kirk Session Records 1697–1828* (Scottish Record Society, Edinburgh, 1968).
11 Rosalind Mitchison, review of James Scott Marshall, *Calendar in Scottish Historical Review LIX* (1970), p. 116.
12 T.C. Smout, 'Scottish Marriage, Regular and Irregular', pp. 204–36. See also R.B. Outhwaite, *Clandestine Marriage in England, 1500–1850* (London & Rio Grande, 1995).
13 'Claverhouse', *Irregular Border Marriages* (Edinburgh, 1934), Chs. 1 and 2.
14 NLS Adv.MS 34–7–9. We are indebted to Tristram Clarke for this reference.
15 Dorothy Leadbeater, 'Problems of Marriage Registration in Scotland, 1700–1855' (unpublished MA thesis, Edinburgh University, 1973), p. 8.
16 A legal collection includes cases from the early nineteenth century where certificates of proclamation had been bought in Parliament Close, in one case for half a guinea. These could then be presented to a Mr Joseph Robertson (later described as a convict) in Leith Wynd Chapel, who would marry the couple. In one case in court in 1818, the acting session clerk stated that only one in 50 of those allegedly 'proclaimed' would actually have been proclaimed. James Fergusson, *Treatise on the Present State of Consistorial Law in Scotland* (Edinburgh, 1829), p. 61.
17 Baptism is the ceremony by which a child first enters the Christian Church. In a period where the Christian congregation and secular society were the same people, and their rules of conduct were congruent, membership of one reinforced membership of the other. Thus baptism conferred secular respectability. It also calmed superstitious fears: in north-east Scotland and the Borders unbaptised children were seen as likely to haunt their parents. J.M. McPherson, *Primitive Beliefs in the North East of Scotland* (London, 1929), pp. 113–14.
18 See the examples quoted in Chapter 3 and *Edinburgh Evening Courant,* 28 October 1758.

5

Patterns in Illegitimacy and Pre-marital Conceptions

Our original aim was to measure the level of illegitimacy in Scotland, and in the various regions, over time. Of particular interest were the south west and north east, where illegitimacy was high in the nineteenth century and indeed into the twentieth.[1] We then found that there were other aspects of sexual behaviour which could be measured: the level of repeated bastard bearing and of premarital pregnancy, and the readiness of the fathers of illegitimate children to admit responsibility and provide support.

As explained in earlier chapters, we confined ourselves to the period between 1660 and 1780 and identified ten regions within Scotland with different social or economic systems. Using the kirk session registers of the parishes which could provide long runs of material we collected the cases of unmarried pregnancy and of births unsuitably soon after the marriage of the parents.[2] The kirk session acted as a court, and demanded unmistakable evidence in the cases that came before it. It was unusual for couples to be caught undeniably in the act of sex, and usually there would just be evidence of 'scandalous carriage'. It was only a pregnancy or birth that was proof positive.

An unmarried woman would be noted in her neighbourhood as presenting a changed shape, a different silhouette. The local elder might notice this himself, or hear the gossip. He would 'delate', that is report, to the session, which would summon the woman to attend and be questioned. If she denied pregnancy, which many did, she would be summoned again. Eventually her pregnancy would become undeniable, whereupon the details would be investigated, including the man responsible. He in turn would be summoned and questioned. The birth of the child or the admission of the mother was proof of fornication and the session would impose its penalty on both parties, a fine and a series of public appearances as penitent on the 'pillar' or 'cutty stool'. Sometimes a woman or couple came to the session to confess.

In order to compute levels of illegitimacy, we had to decide which births within a particular kirk session would be counted as illegitimate. Inevitably these closely follow the definitions used by the kirk sessions themselves:

1 We attributed illegitimate births to the parish where the couples made their penitential appearances, despite where the child was born. Normally kirk sessions confined their disciplinary activity to cases where they believed the intercourse had taken place in the parish.
2 We have not counted as illegitimate any case where the couple was already proclaimed for marriage or where a marriage contract had been signed, as the

5: Patterns in Illegitimacy and Pre-marital Conceptions

child would probably have been born after the marriage. (They would count amongst 'antenuptial' cases, which are discussed later in this chapter.)
3 We have not counted any case where the mother was a married woman, even when the father was definitely not her husband, since the child would not be legally defined as a bastard.
4 We have assumed that when a case led to public appearance in church for fornication (as opposed to scandalous carriage) it definitely resulted in an illegitimate birth.[3]
5 We have recorded twins only where the register makes explicit reference to a double birth. Since details of this kind are sometimes omitted, and since not all births occurred during the period of kirk session investigation, some multiple births will have been counted as single.
6 When it was reported that a mother had 'parted with the child', the phrase used for a miscarriage, we have not counted a birth. We did count every child brought to term, even if reported as born dead, as we have no reliable way of distinguishing between a stillbirth, a child dying almost immediately after birth, and infanticide.

We also had to make rules governing our compilation of time series. Cases were assigned to the year of first mention; the calendar year in Scotland started in January. If registers had big gaps within a year we did not collect for that year. Registers were usually written up or dictated by the minister, and gaps would indicate illness, death or translation to another parish. Sessions might leave discipline to be carried out by a new minister, or keep records only on slips of paper which might get lost or misplaced. So when a register showed no meetings for several months we left that year out of our sample. We collected our figures by decades to smooth out annual fluctuations, and where the record was missing for part of a decade we set the minimum for inclusion of the decade at six years of record.

Of course, it is meaningless to show that one locality had five illegitimate births and another had fifty unless this can be related to the size of the population. Here we had some difficulty. The ideal denominator figure would be the number of unmarried local women of childbearing age (conventionally, fifteen to 45); the number of illegitimate births per thousand such women is the 'illegitimacy rate'. Unfortunately, we have no reliable way of estimating the unmarried population in our period. However, an estimation of total births allows a calculation of the 'illegitimacy ratio', the percentage of births that were illegitimate.

Therefore, the next step in our inquiry was to find or deduce a figure for the average annual number of births in a parish. We used as figures for the parishes' population those produced by the Reverend Alexander Webster in his 'census' of 1755. Webster collected his figures from the minister of each parish; he is believed to have conducted his inquiry carefully, and his figures are as sound as any at that period could be.[4] No reliable figures exist for Scotland's population before Webster's, but it is believed to have grown very slowly in the seventeenth century, to have declined abruptly in the famine of the 1690s, and then risen slowly again. Before the agrarian changes which began in the 1760s the number of householders in a parish was fairly static, except for disaster periods, because it related to specific economic slots in the process of extracting a living from the land by processes which changed very slowly. So we used Webster's figures for the population of our parishes between 1660 and 1780, for part of which period they cannot be more than a

Girls in Trouble

rough guide.

The Webster age distribution figures were used in Flinn's *Scottish Population History* to give a birth rate of 41.6 per thousand, but this figure is now felt to be much too high. A later handling of Webster's age distribution has produced a birth rate of a little under 35 per thousand, which is in line with estimates for England between the 1660s and 1770s, of between 30 and 36 per thousand.[5]

Fortunately, there is also another important source of demographic information for the later eighteenth century, the *Statistical Account of Scotland,* generally known as the *OSA*. The *OSA* was a huge questionnaire survey of every parish minister in Scotland in the 1790s, compiled by Sir John Sinclair. The questionnaires seem to have been completed very conscientiously, and the survey achieved almost 100 per cent return. One of the questions was the annual average of births, and many ministers provided this information not only for the 1790s but for earlier decades as well. We collected the figures for the parishes in our various regions and averaged them. They are probably slightly too low, for ministers are unlikely to have allowed for deaths between birth and baptism for periods when they were not in the parish. However the interval before baptism was very short before the 1770s, so it is only in that decade that the shortfall is likely to be of any significance.[6]

Table 5.1 provides an example of the method used.

Table 5.1: Sample Calculation – Central Lowlands 1761–1770
Four parishes have informative records for this period

	Years recorded	Illegitimacy cases	Population	Expected births
Muiravonside	10	11	1539	477
Logie	8	11	1985	492
Muthill	7	11	2902	630
Fossoway	10	20	1765	547
		53		2146

- Illegitimacy cases counted from KSR by rules described earlier
- Population derived from Webster's census
- Regional birth rate of 31/1000 population/year derived from OSA
- Then, e.g. for Logie, 1985 people and 8 years should have 1.985 x 31 x 8 = 492.23 births
- Total births for the four parishes = 2146 and 53 of them illegitimate so
- Illegitimacy ratio = 2.47%

Using this method, we found that illegitimacy ratios for Scotland as a whole started out at 5 per cent, declining to a low of 3 per cent by 1720, and perhaps rising a little thereafter. That means that the main increase came after our study period, associated with the periods of agricultural and industrial revolution in Scotland.[7] The overall Scottish levels are actually remarkably even.

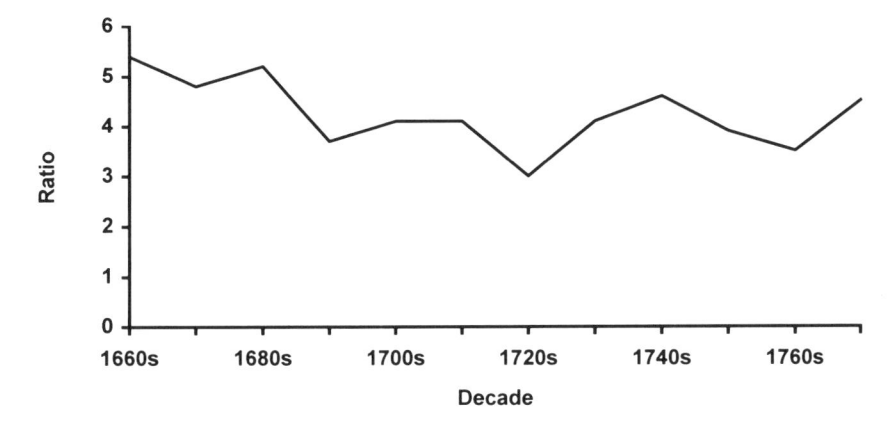

5: Patterns in Illegitimacy and Pre-marital Conceptions

Figure 5.1: Scottish illegitimacy ratios: national sample

These ratios for our period are, however, consistently higher than those for England, until the 1750s when the English figures accelerate and overtake them.[8] What this means is that Scotland, in spite of its strong social regulation of sexual activity, and its strict supervision by presbyteries, from 1660 to 1750 always had proportionally more illegitimacy than England.

The national ratio however conceals a regional diversity, such as a sharp rise in the south-west to some extent cancelled out by falls in the highlands and northern counties. This diversity was one of the starting points for our study, and it is interesting to compare the nineteenth century regional pattern with that pertaining towards the end of our period.

Table 5.2: Illegitimacy ratios: 1760s and 1858–1860

	1760s	1858–60
Lothians	1.0	7.3
Fife	1.8	5.4
Central Lowlands	2.5	8.2
Eastern Highlands	4.0	7.5
Western Highlands	3.9	8.2
Aberdeenshire	3.5	13.7
North-east	4.9	12.1
Caithness	7.6	7.3
Ayrshire	4.8	8.8
South-west	6.1	14.6
Whole country	3.6	9.5

From selected parishes (the same parishes were used for both periods)

Girls in Trouble

Whilst there has been a considerable overall rise, there is also a striking persistence in regional rank order. The Lothians and Fife rank low at both dates, Ayrshire and the highlands occupy a middle position, and the south-west and north-east remain high. The two regions that conspicuously change rank are Caithness and Aberdeenshire.

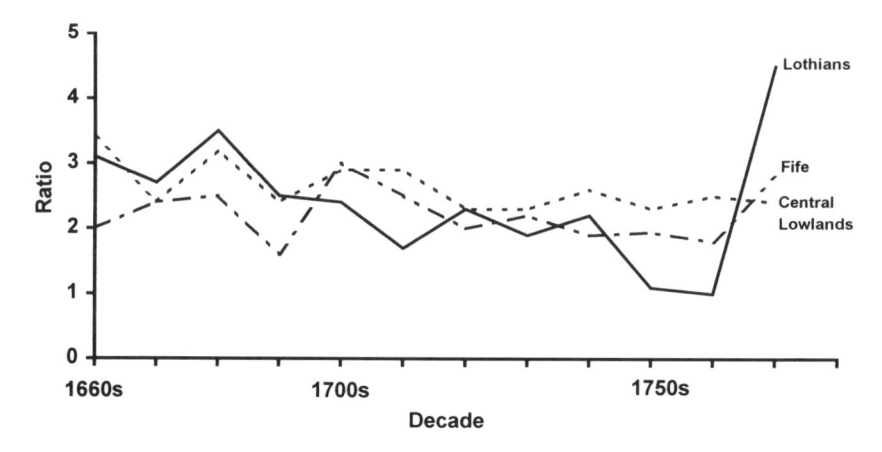

Figure 5.2: Illegitimacy ratios: Lothians, Fife and Central Lowlands

Figure 5.2 shows that illegitimacy was consistently low – below 3 per cent – in the south-east, where the Church's authority was strong. There was however a sharp upturn in the Lothians in the 1770s; we cannot be sure of its significance as the study could not continue into the 1780s and beyond.

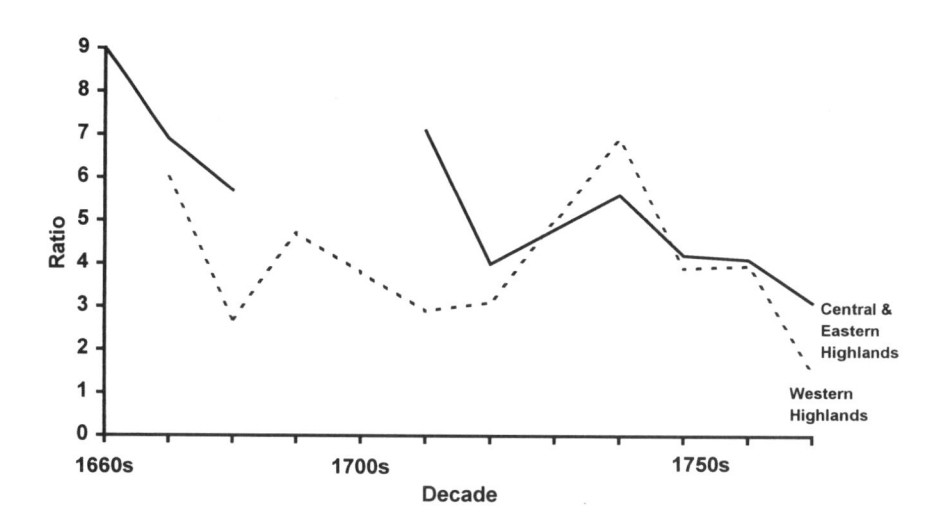

Figure 5.3: Illegitimacy ratios: Western Highlands, Central and Eastern Highlands

5: Patterns in Illegitimacy and Pre-marital Conceptions

Figure 5.3, for the Highlands, has gaps where source material is lacking, but shows a generally high level falling with time. For instance in the Western Highlands illegitimacy ranged from 3 per cent to 6 per cent, and only in the last decade did it drop significantly lower.

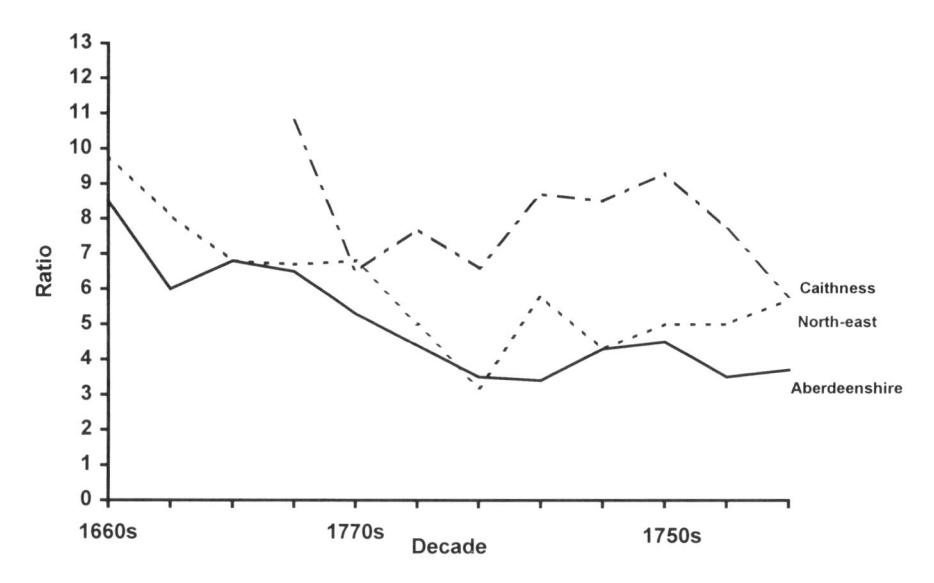

Figure 5.4: Illegitimacy ratios: Aberdeenshire, the North-east and Caithness

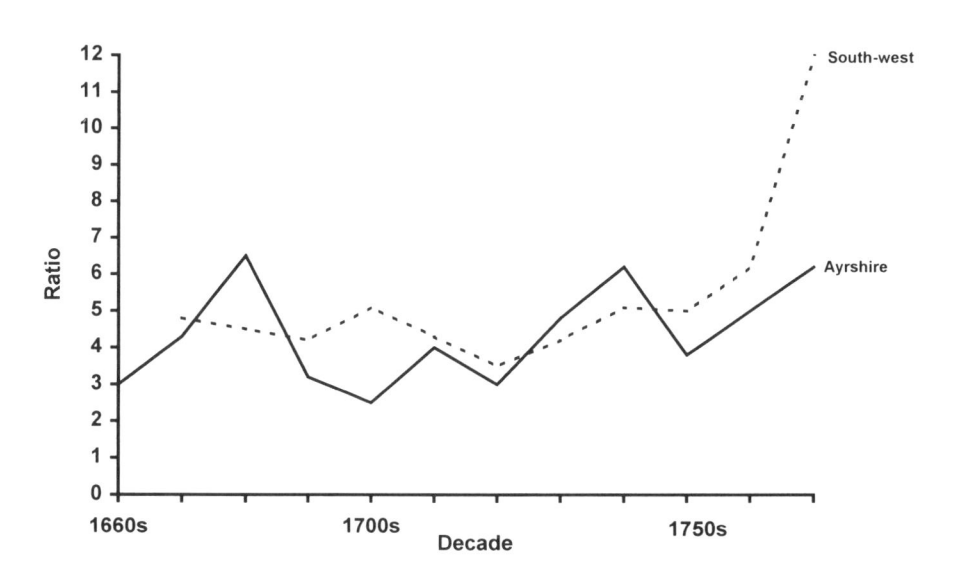

Figure 5.5: Illegitimacy ratios: Ayrshire and the South-west

77

Girls in Trouble

Figure 5.4 shows a downward trend for the north, taking in Aberdeenshire, Caithness and the north-east corner. The fall is from over 8 per cent to around 4 per cent. By contrast, the south-western counties of Dumfriesshire and Galloway, and Ayrshire (Figure 5.5), stay at 4 per cent for most of the period, but with a steep rise from the 1750s. Indeed the rise in the south-west is the main contributor to the slight national rise of that era. (The rise in decadal levels for Ayrshire and the south-west was so marked that we calculated the illegitimacy ratios of the relevant parishes and worked out seven year moving averages; those demonstrated that the averages were not influenced by the divisions between decades but represented a genuine trend.)

Parishes that appear atypical can be identified. Those with notably high illegitimacy ratios include Forglen (north-east), Dailly (Ayrshire), Kilmartin (Western Highlands) and Kemnay (Aberdeenshire). By contrast Kilbirnie (Western Highlands) was low. Alvie (Eastern Highlands), which had high ratios in the nineteenth century, was also higher for the three decades for which its register could be used. The parish with the consistently high level of illegitimacy was Westerkirk in the south-west.

Table 5.3: Illegitimacy ratios: Westerkirk and the South-west

	Westerkirk	South-west
1691–1700	11.2	4.3
1701–10	5.1	9.3
1711–20	4.3	15.1
1721–30	3.6	5.6
1731–40	4.1	9.8

Westerkirk was an upland rural parish, large in area but with a population of only 544 according to Webster. Ratios of 5 per cent, 10 per cent or 15 per cent simply reflect the difference between one, two or three illegitimate births there per year. It was, however, a difference maintained over several decades, and a shadow of it continued into the 1850s, with a level of 18.4 per cent when the south-west regional figure was 14.5 per cent. The minister of a nearby parish, Wamphray, who remarked in the OSA that 'virtuous men are more frequent in the walks of agriculture, than anywhere else' does not seem to have cast about for his evidence.[9] It is not hard to imagine how, in a particular community, bastard-bearing might be perpetuated. There might be certain women who were prolific; over time an extended family would build up with its network of childminding and other support for its unmarried mothers. Thus, without any weakening of the formal constraints as expressed by the kirk session, a counter-culture of illegitimacy could be established.[10]

To test these ideas, we studied the cases which were 'repeaters' – always noted by the kirk session because of the enhanced penalties laid down for these. Some women had a second, third, or fourth illegitimate child, or even more. Overall, between 5 and 15 per cent of all cases of illegitimacy were repeaters. The figures are small and consequently give very variable percentages, but most regions saw a peak around 1700, and Fife and the south-west also peaked in the 1750s. The general trend was down, except in Central Lowlands where it rose, and in the north-east (including also

5: Patterns in Illegitimacy and Pre-marital Conceptions

Aberdeenshire and Caithness) it was consistently higher than elsewhere in the country.

There is no correlation between repeaters and illegitimacy levels in any of our regions, though it is noteworthy that the low level of repeaters in the 1720s and 1730s coincided with the period when church discipline was at its most effective.

These figures are markedly lower than those collected for various English parishes, which range from 7 to 35 per cent. (Relatively few such parishes were studied, so the higher figures may be atypical.) David Levine sees a link between the highest figures and burgeoning intensive cottage-based production of textiles. But in Scotland during the 1760s and 1770s the repeater figure was falling. Laslett has claimed for England that since repeaters were more mobile than other women, some of them may not have been traced. This would not apply to Scotland, for Church detective work was very efficient. Also, our figures do not support his claim that 'a rise in illegitimacy beyond a certain point is no longer a rise in the number of women who have bastards, but rather in the number of bastards borne by a minority of them'.[11]

Did repeaters arise from stable (albeit irregular) unions or from more transient affairs? In every one of the ten regions we found that those pregnant by a different man far outnumbered those pregnant by the same man. There was also a third component, of 'unknowns', that makes it impossible to quantify absolutely, but the consistency of the evidence is unmistakable. To quote the figures from two very different regions: in Ayrshire out of a total of 84 repeaters, 23 were with the same man, 39 were with different men and 22 were untraceable: in the north-east out of a total of 160, 42 were with the same man, 62 with a different man and 56 untraceable. Long standing unions were more easily traced and transgressors identified than for more casual unions, so we are confident that few of the 'unknowns' were quasi-marital relationships; most will have involved liaisons with different men. And even the stable couples, when cited for fornication, did not claim to be 'married'.

The lack of correlation between repeating and overall illegitimacy means that we have found no evidence of an illegitimate counter-culture or the 'bastardy-prone sub-society' postulated by Laslett, at least at regional level. It could still have existed at local level, in particular parishes like Westerkirk. The surname structure of many areas in Scotland, and the lack of certain types of parish record which might provide personal detail, prevent us pursuing this theme.

Another aspect of illegitimacy is the maintenance of the children. Morison's *Dictionary of Decisions* includes some instances of this. In the case of Robert Oliver, a Roxburghshire day labourer, and Janet Scott, a woman of similar rank, in 1778, the man was deemed liable for support of the child until it reached seven, at which point he could either assume custody or continue support until the child was ten. In the case of Agnes Paterson, another woman 'of low rank', the man was ordered to pay 100 pounds Scots (£8.6s.8d sterling) a year until the child was seven. In this case it was argued, but not accepted, that a boy would be earning at seven and a girl at ten.[12]

Most cases concerning child maintenance which came before kirk sessions did not involve the propertied class. In the earliest that we found (Alves, December 1661), a specific sum was not mentioned, but William Forsyth 'became willingly enacted and obliged to maintaine according to his abilitie & state of lyfe, the child called Issobell Forsyth procreated between him and Janet Stenner in fornication'. A cautioner was produced to ensure he fulfilled his obligation, and the session appointed an extract of the act to be given to the woman, 'that if the said William fails in performance

79

according to his undertaking, she may have recourse to the Session for redress & assistance'. In another seventeenth-century case (Trinity Gask, September 1674), the minister reported that Janet Wedderspoon had come to him saying that Thomas Wandles, the father of her child, 'will give her nothing for the bairns maintenance and she has nothing to nourish him with'. The man appeared before the session '& affirmed that for the present he had nothing to give her, but after harvest what he might spare of his fie should be given to her'. The session told the woman of the man's promise, '& knowing her indigence they appoynt for her weeklie two shilling scots during this harvest'.

In the eighteenth century there appears to have been some standardisation in the amount payable. We discovered two cases concerning child maintenance in Kenmore (August 1733 and June 1736) and in both of them the man was expected to bear the expense of half the child's board. That this was not just a local custom is attested in a case which appears in Morison's *Dictionary of Decisions* for 1758: a woman had got a Justice of the Peace decision that the man should provide half the child's maintenance (50 shillings a year) until the age of ten.[13]

However, the standardisation of responsibility cannot have been universal, or there would have been no need for Alexander Fletcher and Janet McGrigor to have come before Kenmore session (December 1759) and agree to abide by the session's decision regarding the maintenance of their two bastard children.

> The session after considering the affair ordain that for the two years and three quarters she has had the eldest child The said Alexander shall pay unto her fourty pounds scots money including thirty five shillings sterling which she acknowledges to have received already in part payment for said time for maintaining & cloathing the said eldest Child: and that in all time coming Alexr shall keep & maintain said Child without any trouble or expense to the mother: The session further ordain, that as to maintaining the youngest child, Alexander shall pay unto said Janet eight pounds scots, quarter about, for nursing & maintaining said youngest Child till he be six quarters old, after which time she the mother obliges herself to maintain & cloth her said youngest Child in all time coming without any trouble or expence of the father.

Although the mother of a bastard child might at times receive charity, sessions felt no obligation to maintain bastard children. In Wemyss (April and June 1704), the session was informed that Margaret Hill, whose partner had fled, 'hath absented this paroch and hath left her child with a nourse which hath been burdensom to the session already'. A search was made for the woman, the Church espionage system was as efficient as usual, and she was found. The session asked her to explain her actions. She insisted she had planned to return, but that 'whither present or absent she was not able to pay for the mentinance of her child. The child with the nourse being present the child was delivered to its mother and she was told in plain terms she behoved to go work for a mentinance to herself and child & not be any longer burdensome or troublesome to the Session'.

The readiness of fathers to support their illegitimate children is discussed in Chapter 7. The surprisingly high level of men accepting responsibility means that one argument about Scottish illegitimacy in the nineteenth century, that it reflected the ease with which a woman could find work and so support herself and her child, is of limited relevance in this period.

5: Patterns in Illegitimacy and Pre-marital Conceptions

Ostensibly the Church made no distinction of rank or class. The women who bore bastards were, like most of the population, in simple manual occupations. The most common occupation recorded was 'servitrix' which might indicate domestic service, but could also cover work on a farm or servant to a craftsman. In over seven thousand cases we came across only a handful of women of higher status. Women of rank or property may have been more virtuous than working women, or, very probably, were better protected and guarded. Such women were of value because property could be redistributed by their marriages. By contrast the men in our cases came from all ranks. Often they were fellow servants in the same household, but masters and masters' sons were frequently sexually involved with servants. Such men were not necessarily of higher status, for it was common for the young of both sexes, when old enough to start working, to be placed as servants in the households of near kin. There were also men of higher rank in our sample, and these were resistant to Church discipline. Some might be ready to support an illegitimate child, but there were strong objections to undergoing 'appearances' (see Chapter 7).

We have now presented our figures and looked at different aspects of illegitimacy but have not yet advanced theories or explanations. If we want to explain illegitimacy ratios in Scotland between 1660 and 1780, that explanation is going to have to account for some marked differences in time, by region, and by contrast with England. Of course, it could be argued that the figures we have collected contain too many statistical uncertainties for meaningful analysis. We are aware of the imperfections in our methods, but though they may well apply at parish level, for an individual decadal figure, and for part of the difference with eighteenth-century England and nineteenth-century Scotland, they cannot begin to account for the regional and temporal patterns we have found. In seeking to understand our illegitimacy ratios it may be helpful to look at categories of explanation which have been advanced for other cultures and time periods.

One such category is connected with fertility. The people of this period had no reliable contraception or abortion. There may have been some changes in fertility: a well-fed and disease-free people will reach sexual maturation earlier, and are more likely to have sex result in pregnancy. Such changes in population health however are more likely to be reflected in overall fertility rates and in infant mortality, which we could not study, and to have little effect on illegitimacy ratios (as opposed to rates). Moreover, there was no major change of that kind in this period, other than the famine years after 1690.

A second category focuses on the economic system. For example, did work patterns segregate the sexes or bring them together, did it promote mobility and financial freedom or was it exploitive, what was the economic plight of the unmarried mother, and so on. In many ways this is tied in with the question of social control; a system that encouraged young people to enter service in other households might in isolation have promoted promiscuity and illegitimacy, but in these circumstances it did not. For the Lothians we found that some 5 per cent to 10 per cent of the men were fellow servants, and 5 per cent to 20 per cent were masters or sons of masters, a percentage lower than those found in a similar analysis by Keith Wrightson for seventeenth-century Essex, though similar to Lancashire.[14]

The rise in English illegitimacy, especially from 1740 to 1780, has been linked to proto-industrialisation; the growth of 'cottage industry', transitional between the independent artisan and mass mill production. In Scotland no industry rivalled linen, which grew rapidly in the 1740s and 1750s, for the work opportunities and income offered to young people. But linen was most conspicuous in eastern Scotland, much less so in Galloway and the south-west where illegitimacy ratios were rising. The biggest long-term economic change, the movement into the cities, by definition cannot be assessed by a study confined to rural parts, but it only became a major force in the closing years of our period. Overall then, we do not discount economic explanations, but cannot see an obvious correlation with illegitimacy.

Another category of explanations relate to customs and controls around marriage, rather than around sexuality. For example, there is the argument that the official definition of marriage, and hence of children born outside it, was not the same as the popular one. Such a system can, for instance, be seen in eighteenth-century Sweden.[15] As we have seen in Chapter 4, an irregular marriage was still a legal marriage in Scotland, and (as noted earlier when discussing 'repeaters') couples cited for fornication did not claim to be irregularly married, unless they could produce a certificate to prove it.

The idea of 'fertility testing' – that a man would be unwilling to marry a woman until she had demonstrated her ability to bear a child – is still remarkably prevalent outside academic circles. But it is difficult to see a motive, e.g. in land rights or child labour, and in any case this would lead to bridal pregnancy rather than illegitimacy.

Another theory, first posited by Peter Laslett, is that of interrupted or frustrated courtship: expectations of some couples of being able to marry would be destroyed by social and economic events, and the result would be the pregnancy of an unmarried woman. Support for this idea for early modern England is based on the fact that the average age at which an unmarried mother gave birth corresponded closely to that of married woman at the birth of their first child.[16] But this would imply a much higher level of pre-marital pregnancy than existed in our period.

Certainly it was expected that couples should be in a position to support a family before they married. Some states of South Germany in the nineteenth century adopted Malthusian dogmas and denied marriage to the poor, with consequent high illegitimacy rates.[17] In late nineteenth-century Banffshire it was frequently alleged that deliberate restrictions on cottage building by the farmers had an important role in the high levels of illegitimacy.[18] But no such restraints – whether official or unofficial – were found in any of our regions during our period.

What emerged most strongly in the course of our research was the link between illegitimacy and church control. The argument becomes circular if low levels of illegitimacy are cited as proof of effective control, but the only symptom of this control is the low illegitimacy. The argument needs corroborating by other indicators, and the acid test is provided by the highlands, where illegitimacy fell, and the south-west, where it rose markedly. In the highlands there can be no doubt that the early part of this period was turbulent, and neither the Church nor any other central authority could hold sway, but that discipline became more surely founded by the end of the seventeenth century. A late nineteenth-century commentator noted about the kirk session:

> Of all judicatories it was the most respected and best obeyed; for the Highlanders, remiss and careless in other matters, set great store by the ordinances of baptism and communion; and the cutty-stool and sackcloth gown were much more dreaded in 1700 than the threats of law and 'tout' of the royal horn. Seeing there were few restrictions on the intercourse of the sexes, and considering the oblique idea they

5: Patterns in Illegitimacy and Pre-marital Conceptions

had of some other moral duties, it is astonishing to find how little the evil of illegitimacy prevailed.[19]

Retrospective comments like this are easily made, and can prove quite wrong. More convincing is the increasing success of the church in establishing its ministers, and holding sessional courts at all, in highland areas.

In the whole north-eastern and northern areas the picture is different. Northern Scotland had, on the whole, taken a different political line from the south in the disturbances of the seventeenth century. In particular, the north-east and Aberdeenshire had supported episcopacy, and consequently suffered severe dislocation after the Revolution of 1689, when the General Assembly expelled ministers who had accepted episcopacy, often on trumped up charges, and intruded presbyterians in their place. It would be surprising if the attachment to the court system of presbyterianism was as strong here as in the south.

The unusual pattern of illegitimacy in the south-west also correlates with a high level of resistance to church discipline. In the south-west men were much tardier in admitting responsibility for a pregnancy, and in Ayrshire and the south-west together less than half of the men named made a rapid admission, whereas elsewhere the 'admission rate' was usually over two-thirds (see Chapter 7). One man in the south-west even refused to take the oath disclaiming adultery, and protested about the discipline system to the highest court in the Church, the Commission of the General Assembly. His particular ground for resistance was the low social standing of the woman who had named him. The synod, to which the affair had also gone, did not share his sense of social superiority and considered that he was an undesirable example of the men who got girls into trouble and then deserted them: 'Poor women are decoyed by Men into Uncleanness', stated the synod adding, 'Men accused do usually deny and refuse to give Oath' but 'are prepared everywhere to acknowledge guilt except before a Church judicatory'.[20] In the south-west such men were often aided by the women, who would refuse to give names. There was also in these two regions a high proportion of cases where the women ran away rather than face discipline. It is interesting that Galloway, the base area of irreconcilable Covenanting sentiment and the only area of militant Lowland resistance to agricultural improvement, should have resisted the sexual discipline of the Church.

Another form of sexual misbehaviour recorded by the kirk session was 'antenuptial fornication', revealed by pregnancy predating the marriage.[21] Any birth within nine calendar months of the marriage would lead to a thorough investigation, and until the matter was settled, either by acquittal of the parents or by their penance, baptism would be denied the child. The use of calendar months ignored some simple facts: first, that months are of different lengths, and a nine-month term can vary in length by as much as three days. Second, gestation should be timed from the menstrual cycle, not the date of intercourse. In any case, some births occur early.[22]

For this reason it is preferable only to count births within eight months of marriage as those most probably conceived out of wedlock. However, our material does not allow this, since old parish registers (OPRs) in Scotland often record not the date of marriage but the date of proclamation. It does, however, allow us to draw upon the suspicions of the local community. The parish investigation would be thoroughly conducted and thoroughly recorded, though it is bound to miss some out of wedlock pregnancies that came late to term.

Girls in Trouble

In spite of a General Assembly ruling that antenuptial fornicators should receive the same punishment whether they subsequently married or did not,[23] parishes did not set a uniform penalty, and sessions used their discretion. In Thurso (June 1692) James Bain had sworn he was not guilty of antenuptial fornication, but when his child was born it was found 'by computation' that the child had been begotten before he took this oath. This was regarded as a heinous sin, and he had to appear in sackcloth. In the case of William Moody in Forgandenny (January 1750) 'in regard the scandall was flagrant in the parish long before their marriage, the session were of opinion that both he and his wife aught to satisfie in the same way as all other ordinary fornicators being persuaded that nothing less could tend to Edification in their Case'. Conversely, Longside session decided that as James Davidson and Jean Rennet (March 1773) 'had been married before the Scandal became flagrant' it was sufficient to rebuke them privately instead of publicly.

As an extra weapon in the fight for good behaviour sessions came to demand 'consignation money' from couples when they put their names down to be proclaimed for marriage. The money would be returned if nine months elapsed before a child was born.[24] Another ploy if there was any doubt about a possible premarital conception, was for the minister to grant baptism of a first child only on condition that the father provided a cautioner that he and his wife would satisfy discipline if it should turn out that they had been guilty of antenuptial fornication.

Most sessions came to regard 'antenuptial uncleanness' as less reprehensible than straightforward fornication in spite of the ruling of the General Assembly. The usual penalty by the mid-eighteenth century was one appearance and half the normal fine. Wemyss (Fife) stood out for a long time against such leniency. The minister in August 1752 suggested inflicting 'a lesser Censure' on 'those who committed uncleanness before they married one another than on others who did not marry those they committed uncleanness with'. The session refused. It was not until June 1769 that the session, aware of 'the complaint that has been often made to them that their Discipline as to Antenuptial Fornication is severer than in all neighbouring Parishes & considering that it was not well proportion'd to have those who marry and those who marry not upon an equal footing', fell in line with others and allowed a rebuke.

The share of antenuptial conceptions in total births was surprisingly low in all regions, and particularly so – under 1 per cent – in Caithness, where illegitimacy was relatively high. In Ayrshire it rose above 2 per cent for the 1740s and 1760s, and in Fife for the 1700s; otherwise in all regions it was well below 2 per cent. Fife shows a close relationship between the illegitimacy ratio and the antenuptial conceptions. (Many illegitimate births there occurred not because the couple failed to marry but because they did it too late. The Church realistically treated these cases as antenuptial fornication.) The figures in most regions show little relationship to the figures for illegitimacy. At a national level the share was about 1 per cent.

The problem with these figures is that the denominator is total births, whereas it is the proportion of *first* births that is the better indicator. Unfortunately, only one Scottish OPR provides sufficient information to derive this figure, and that is Kilmarnock. If we use this one parish as a rough guide for the whole of Scotland, then approximately a quarter of births were the mothers' first.

As a proportion of first births the trends in antenuptial conceptions clarify and show a distinct trend. Nationally, they rise from just over three per cent of first births in the 1660s to nearly five per cent in the 1770s, with regional variations. In Fife, the

5: Patterns in Illegitimacy and Pre-marital Conceptions

Central Lowlands and Lothian the trend is markedly downward; in the north-east and Aberdeenshire it is upward; in the highlands and Caithness there is no obvious trend; in Ayrshire and the south-west the trend is upwards from the 1720s.

Nearly half of these antenuptial conceptions were known to the kirk session before the marriage, but, there was considerable variation in the alertness of the elders, with the Eastern Highlands and the north-east being quickest in discovery.

Table 5.4: Time of discovery of antenuptial conception (%)

	Before marriage	Between marriage and birth	After birth
Lothians	31	9	60
Fife	36	13	51
Central Lowlands	56	9	35
Eastern Highlands	74	9	17
Western Highlands	25	14	61
Aberdeenshire	59	14	27
North-east	70	6	25
Caithness	42	10	48
Ayrshire	42	19	40
South-west	39	12	49
All regions	47	11	42

That relatively few were pursued between marriage and birth is understandable, since all sessions would be bound to check the date of marriage at the time of the birth.

In some cases enough information was given to the session to enable it to date the conception. In three quarters of these cases the marriage took place between the fifth and the eighth month of pregnancy. Some couples may have believed that either betrothal or proclamation, both regarded as part of the marriage process, was equivalent to marriage. Sometimes the gap between these preliminaries and marriage might be considerable. In May 1676 Wemyss session declared that 'divers persones in this parishe after they give up their names for mariadge, Delayes the same verie long and comitts fornication between Contract and mariadge'. In August 1675 a Dalkeith couple confessed antenuptial fornication but said 'it was after purpose and paction of marriage'. In Wemyss, January 1704, John Brown and Isabel Davidson, 'being asked when they were guilty answered the same night they were contracted'. In Kinglassie, January 1759, George Aitkin, whose first child was born seven months after marriage, denied fornication. A week later 'he declar'd that by refusing antenuptial Guilt he only meant to refuse guilt before marriage in his heart and did not deny that he was guilty with Margaret Taylor before the proclamation of Banns and publick celebration of his marriage with her'.

Some sessions considered fornication between contract and marriage to be a less heinous sin. In Kinglassie (September 1724) John Baxter asked to be let off with only one appearance since he was going to marry the woman involved. This the session would not allow, 'it being Reported that the woman was with Child before

Girls in Trouble

Contract of marriage'. In Kenmore (September 1754) the session dismissed a couple with only a sessional, not a public, rebuke, 'in regard the Guilt was Committed between Contract and marriage.'

The rigid (and somewhat inaccurate) way of calculating the gestation must have caused anxiety in many a newly wed couple. The minister of Penpont in 1694 recorded in his memoir about his recently acquired wife:

> all the time her being with child I was still afraid lest she a very young lass, being but yet in her 19 year through her rashness or carelessness of herself, should bring forth before the due time, which made me put my request... often to God... that so he might not open the mouths of the Ungodly.[25]

There was no kirk session enquiry or comment by the ungodly because in the event the couple had 25 hours on the side of respectability, but the minister's fears provide an insight into the ethos of his day.

Inevitably, there were early births where a couple denied having had premarital sex. The usual procedure in such cases was for a midwife to pronounce on whether the child was premature or 'ripe', and innocent reasons for an early birth might also be accepted. For example, when Marion Ron (Logie, February 1697) gave birth six weeks early, it was said that she 'had got a fall when she was with Child and was never well again after that fall till she was brought to bed', and the session dropped the case. In Wemyss (August 1709), the child of Bernard Walker and Margaret Walker was born 27 days early, and they denied guilt. The man declared 'it was very well known she had got a stress which made her bring forth her child before the time'. The session clearly did know of this, and knew furthermore that there had been no reports of scandalous carriage between them, and therefore agreed to baptise the child. (However, it still insisted on the man's binding himself to satisfy discipline if evidence later came to light which proved him guilty.)

The testimony of midwives was not considered infallible. In Canisbay (August 1714) William Howet and Christian Rugg craved baptism for their child born eight months after marriage. The minister reported he had had the infant inspected, and 'it was found to have all the signs of a timely birth'. The couple continued denying that they had had premarital intercourse, and there was no other evidence of guilt, so the session referred the case to presbytery and when the couple continued to deny, their innocence was accepted. In Wemyss (March 1730), the child of David Tilloch and Elspeth Brown was born 27 days early. The midwife declared the child 'was as proper & full born as any child she received'. The affair was delayed, and two years later the man approached the minister again, craving baptism. When he continued to deny antenuptial fornication he was asked if he was willing to swear a solemn oath; when he did so the child was baptised.

Solemn oaths were used both in suspected antenuptial fornication cases and in ordinary fornication cases where a man denied paternity. The Church's practice was to allow such an oath to be taken only if it considered that the man was likely to be innocent as claimed. Wemyss session register for August 1673 records such an oath:

> Compeired John Stirling befoir the pulpit and sitting there upon a stoole the whole tyme of the forenoones exercise at the close thereof gave his oath The tenor whereoff follows I Johne Stirling with uplifted hand to heaven Doe declare before the Lord God, the searcher off hearts, As I shall answer to him in the great day,

5: Patterns in Illegitimacy and Pre-marital Conceptions

wherein he shall judge the quick & the dead, And render to every one according to their works, That I never did comitt the act of uncleanness and fornication with Christian Pirie and iff this my declaration be not true, Then let me be seperate from the presence of God for ever, And even in this Life be ane example of Gods vengeance and wroth against all perjurie and uncleannesse.

The vigorous language of this oath appears more effective as an instrument of coercion than the officially recommended version.[26]

Sometimes sessions did not require an oath but simply used their common sense. In Cramond (June 1734) Margaret Fairholm gave birth to a seven month child and denied guilt. 'The session considering that there had been no presumption, save that she had brought forth her child about the seventh month after marriage, which is no extraordinary case; they thought fit to proceed no further in this affair'. In Kingsbarns (July 1747), David Campbell and Alison Lesles denied guilt after the birth of twins four weeks early. The midwife declared that there 'was nothing more ordinary for a woman with twins than to bring them furth in the eight month'; the session allowed baptism to go ahead.

In marked contrast to the attitude of the sessions above, was that shown in a case in Torphichen (May 1727). The session appeared determined to believe the worst. Mrs Tait, 'spouse to Mr John Tait Chyrugeon', gave birth to a child six weeks early. The minister believed the couple innocent and presented various reasons to the session: she had been ill of 'a violent Ague' for several months before she gave birth, she had 'met with a Fright' a few days before delivery, the child could not suck and had no proper nails on some toes etc. However the midwife thought the child was full term and the session therefore insisted on the testimony of several of the women who had attended the birth. All declared they thought the child premature, and Mr Tait solemnly declared his innocence, but the session decided it required further evidence and called more of the women who had attended the birth. It was not until a letter was produced from 'Mrs Forrest' (i.e. Mistress, implying gentry status) which declared her belief in the child being born early that the session allowed baptism to go ahead. In the postscript to the letter Mrs Forrest added: 'I could have wished there had not been so much Din about it, it shews little Love to the Credit of the Gospel to put such Things in the Mouths of the wicked and ignorant'.

There is a further category of women to be looked at: those who were guilty of fornication before marriage but not with the man they married. We did not count the issue of such liaisons as bastards, since by Scots law they were considered legitimate, though the child may well have been stigmatised as a bastard within the community. It was not a common occurrence: out of a total of 1,961 pre-marital conceptions, 31 were known to have been fathered by a man other than the husband. Cases occurred as early as the 1660s and as late as the 1770s, and there was no region which did not have at least one. The highest number, seven, occurred in the Eastern Highlands, four of these in Kenmore parish in the 1740s. In Petty, another Eastern Highlands parish, the session recorded of one woman in 1765 that she was 'with child by antenuptial fornication to her own husband' as though it were a surprise. No particular shock or horror was expressed at a woman bearing her first child to a man not her husband in any of the session minutes of this region.

Indeed, it was surprisingly rare for sessions in *any* of the regions to express any condemnation of such a thing. We found such expressions in only four of the cases, three of them in Ayrshire. In Grange, a north-east parish, in 1717, the session

Girls in Trouble

concluded that Margaret Dason 'was guilty of a remarkable wickedness in marrying with an other man's child in her womb'. The elders were 'difficultyed in passing sentence against her, in regard the like had not happened formerly in this place in their time'. In the first of the Ayrshire cases (Kilmarnock, July 1698), Jannet McClunnochin claimed 'she never knew she was with child unto the said John Muir untill both herself and her husband William Aitken had found it moving and stirring in her belly, and so was removed with indignation at her disingenuity and dissimulation'. In another Ayrshire case (Kilbirnie, November 1760) Jean Sherret, married to John Blain, confessed that the child she brought forth six months after marriage was fathered by Hugh Orr. The session considered this case unusual enough to consult presbytery, and when she was publicly rebuked it was not just for her sin of fornication but also 'for her deceiving the man she was married to, by entering into marriage with him when she was with child to another man'. It is surprising not to find such sentiments expressed more often in such cases.

Somewhat less than a fifth of the women who bore children in our period conceived their first child out of wedlock. This figure is arrived at by taking the total number of fornication cases, removing from it the repeaters, adding on the number disciplined for 'antenuptial uncleanness' and taking the result as a quarter of the estimated annual births in the parishes (based, as before, on the OPRs of Kilmarnock). The total level of such conceptions may seem high, largely because of the component from illegitimacy.

This proportion, expressed as a percentage, varies little, ranging between 16 per cent and 23 per cent, with a slight fall in the seventeenth century, but some regional figures show much greater variation. That for the north-east was over 40 per cent in the 1660s and fell rapidly in the next twenty years, thereafter varying between 14 per cent and 27 per cent. The south-west shows a different trend, starting at 14 and ending at 45. In this, as in other measurements we see the south-west from the 1750s refusing to abide by the conventions. In all regions and periods the major component in the figure is illegitimacy, and so inevitably it mirrors trends discussed earlier. Premarital fornication provided less than one in fifty of annual births, and less than a quarter of the cases of first births conceived out of wedlock.

The relatively static level of first conceptions starting outwith marriage in Scotland contrasts with that shown by Wrigley for England. Wrigley's figures show antenuptial conceptions at about 15 per cent of first births in the late seventeenth century, when a further 1.4 per cent of births were illegitimate, rising to 35 per cent premarital conceptions and 4.8 per cent illegitimate in the 1770s.[27] If family size was similar to that of Kilmarnock somewhere between 50 and 60 per cent of first conceptions took place out of marriage. The marked upward trend of the English figures suggests that intercourse during courtship was becoming normal in the later eighteenth century. This would be an improbable interpretation for Scotland. Only in Fife and Ayrshire do the patterns of premarital conceptions and for illegitimacy follow similar lines and even there the level of unwed conceptions is still low. A more probable interpretation of the Scottish figures is that a fairly constant proportion of couples intending marriage entered on intercourse before marriage, and a separate group, with no immediate prospects of marriage, produced illegitimate children.

5: Patterns in Illegitimacy and Pre-marital Conceptions

Notes

1. For instance, the percentage of illegitimate births for Scotland as a whole in the 1850s was 8.9, but in Banffshire it was 16.0 and in Wigtownshire and the Stewartry of Kirkcudbright 12.1 and 13.8 respectively. By contrast other counties had much lower figure; Ross and Cromarty 8.8, Caithness 7.8, East Lothian 7.7. Individual parishes in the north east and south west had more startling figures: Marnock in Banffshire 21.2, Torthorwald in Dumfriesshire 25.6, Knockando in Moray 28.3. T.C. Smout, 'Sexual behaviour in Nineteenth century Scotland' in Peter Laslett, Karla Osterveen and Richard M. Smith (eds.), *Bastardy and its Comparative History* (London, 1982), p. 200.
2. Part of the quantitative results shown in this chapter have already been published in our paper 'Scottish illegitimacy ratios in the early modern period', *Economic History Review* (2nd series, XL, 1987), pp. 45–63.
3. In some parishes in the seventeenth-century pregnancy was not explicitly referred to, but in the eighteenth century the allegation of fornication would not be made until the woman was visibly pregnant, usually in the sixth or seventh month, and sometimes not until after the birth of the child. Of 1,981 cases of fornication found by Stephen J. Davies in Stirlingshire between 1637 and 1747, only 26 of the women were not pregnant. Stephen J. Davies, 'Law and Order in Stirlingshire 1637–1747' (unpublished PhD thesis, St Andrews University, 1984).
4. J.G. Kyd (ed.), *Scottish Population Statistics* (Scottish History Society, Edinburgh, 1952), gives Webster's census and age distribution. See also M.W. Flinn (ed.), *Scottish Population History from the Seventeenth Century to the 1930s* (Cambridge, 1977), pp. 58–64, 181, 200; R.E. Tyson, 'The Population of Aberdeenshire, 1695–1755: a new approach', *Northern Scotland 6* (1985), pp. 113–31. We would like to thank J. Oeppen of the Cambridge Group for the Study of Population and Social Structure for help in abandoning the Flinn figures from Webster.
5. Rosalind Mitchison, 'Webster Revisited: a re-examination of the "census" of Scotland', in T.M. Devine (ed.), *Improvement and Enlightenment* (Edinburgh, 1988), pp. 62–77; E.A. Wrigley and R.S. Schofield, *The Population History of England: a Reconstruction, 1541–1871* (London, 1981).
6. The main weakness of using our regional base figures is the absence in the OSA of information on the numbers of births within the dissenting congregations. But in our period these congregations mostly used the registers of the established church.
7. A recent study based on the parish of Rothiemay in Banffshire shows that there illegitimacy began to rise towards its remarkably high level of the later nineteenth century only after 1811, though pre-marital pregnancy had begun its upward movement in the 1770s. J.A.D. Blaikie, *Illegitimacy, Sex and Society: North-East Scotland, 1750–1900* (Oxford, 1993), Ch. 3.
8. Laslett, Osterveen and Smith (eds.), *Bastardy and its Comparative History*, p. 14.
9. *OSA xxi* (1797), p. 458 (original edition).
10. An explanation of this type might account for the high level of illegitimacy in a large parish, Terling, in the opening decades of the seventeenth century. See David Levine and Keith Wrightson, 'The social context of illegitimacy in early modern England' in Laslett, Osterveen and Smith (eds.), *Bastardy and its Comparative History*, pp. 158–75.
11. 'Family reconstitution and the study of bastardy from certain English parishes', Introduction to ibid., pp. 86–93. On page 86 Richard Smith writes that it appeared 'that as the bastardy ratio went up the proportion of women producing more than one bastard went up at an even faster pace.' Laslett makes this point also in his *Family Forms and Illicit Love in Earlier Centuries* (Cambridge, 1977), p. 147.
12. W.H. Morison, *The Decisions of the Court of Session... in the form of a Dictionary* (Edinburgh, 1811), vols.1 and 2, pp. 438, 400, 444.
13. Ibid., p. 1357. This case came to court because the woman had married and the man was

demanding that the child be handed over to him; the judgment left her with custody. The pound Scots, used in some of the decisions, was worth a twelfth of the pound sterling.
14. Laslett, Osterveen and Smith (eds.), *Bastardy and its Comparative History*, pp. 187–8. He found that at least 28 per cent of Essex and 8 per cent of Lancashire fathers were fellow servants, and at least 23 per cent of Essex fathers and 14 per cent of Lancashire fathers were in a magisterial position *vis-à-vis* the mothers (masters, masters' kin or gentlemen). He also found that if couples were not actually serving in the same household then they were likely to be neighbours; this is not something which can be easily ascertained for Scotland.
15. David Gaunt, 'Illegitimacy in Seventeenth- and Eighteenth-Century East Sweden', in ibid., pp. 313–26.
16. Peter Laslett, Introduction, in ibid., pp. 1–60. But the work of David Levine, in *Family Formation in an Age of Nascent Capitalism* (New York, 1977), Ch. 9, suggests that this was not general.
17. Patricia James (ed.), *The Travel Diaries of Thomas Robert Malthus* (Cambridge, 1966), pp. 153, 277; Knodel, 'Law, Marriage, and Illegitimacy in Nineteenth-Century Germany', *Population Studies xx* (1966–7), pp. 279–94.
18. Smout, 'Sexual Behaviour', p. 202.
19. D. Campbell, *The Lairds of Glenlyon* (Perth, 1886), p. 113.
20. SRO, CH1/2/85.
21. For late eighteenth-century England Wrigley has shown that some 39 per cent of first legitimate births occurred within eight months of marriage and most of these within six months His conclusion from this is that marriage in Europe should be seen as 'a repertoire of adaptable systems rather than as a single pattern'. E.A. Wrigley, 'Marriage, Fertility and Population Growth in Eighteenth Century England' in R.B. Outhwaite (ed.), *Marriage and Society* (London, 1981), pp. 157, 168. See also P.E.H. Hair, 'Bridal Pregnancy in Rural England in Earlier Centuries', *Population Studies xx*, pp. 233–43 and 'Bridal Pregnancy in Earlier Rural England further examined', *Population Studies xxiv* (1970), pp. 59–76.
22. Men claiming that they were not responsible for a pregnancy held this rigid idea of the length of gestation. Measuring from the time of intercourse was, by the mid-eighteenth century, out of line with medical knowledge. William Smellie, *A Treatise on the Theory and Practice of Midwifery* (London, 1752), Vol. 1, p. 126, gives gestation as 'Nine solar months... from the last discharge'.
23. A. Peterkin, *Records of the Kirk of Scotland, containing the Acts and Proceedings of the General Assemblies* (Edinburgh, 1838), Vol. 1, p. 445.
24. For examples of rulings by kirk sessions see Dalkeith October 1678, Auchterarder July 1684, or Fordyce August 1740.
25. National Library of Scotland MS 3045, Diary of the Rev. James Murray.
26. The official form of oath is given in Walter Steuart, *Collections and Observations Concerning the Worship, Discipline and Government of the Church of Scotland* (Edinburgh, 1773), p. 250. 'I... do declare before God and this... that I am innocent and free of the said sin of... of having carnal knowledge of the said C.D. and hereby call the great God, the judge and avenger of all falsehoods, to be witness and judge against me in this matter if I be guilty; and this I do, by taking his blessed name in my mouth, and swearing by him, who is the great judge, punisher, and avenger as said is, and that in the sincerity of my heart, according to the truth of the matter and my own conscience, as I shall answer to God in the last and great day, when I shall stand before him to answer for all that I do in the flesh, and as I would partake of his glory in heaven after this life is at an end.'
27. Wrigley, 'Marriage, Fertility and Population Growth in Eighteenth-Century England', p. 157.

6

Where, When and Why

The previous chapter summarised the quantitative evidence on illegitimacy in Scotland, but many questions remain that require a different approach. What were the circumstances in which these women became pregnant? Where and when did it occur? Why did it happen: were they raped, expecting the man to marry them, or just succumbing to persuasion or to vigorous courtship? Who were the men who got them pregnant; was it a casual relationship; what were the prospects of marriage; what were the circumstances of the seduction? Fortunately, many kirk session registers went beyond the 'bare bones' of a case and provided us with fuller information. In this chapter we attempt to resolve queries of this nature,[1] though inevitably there are aspects of our subject for which we have no good information. For example, we cannot ascertain whether there were differences in the age of girls falling pregnant, between regions or over time. We have little information on courtship practices other than statements of disapproval, which could have a bearing on illegitimacy levels, as T.C. Smout has shown for the nineteenth century.[2] Nevertheless, such qualitative evidence as we do have gives insight into many of the opening questions.

Previously we stated that an accusation of fornication would normally be made only on the evidence of pregnancy (see Chapter 5). However, kirk session registers also contain many examples of 'scandalous carriage', where a couple was caught in a compromising position. They might, for instance, be alone in a house together with the door barred but not actually caught in the act, and with no ensuing pregnancy to prove their fornication. Such cases often took up an inordinate amount of time because the evidence was circumstantial and witnesses would have to be interrogated. Scandalous carriage was a lesser sin than fornication, but if proven the couple would still be rebuked in front of the congregation.

In Kenmore in the Central Highlands (December 1750), the session heard of a 'clamant Report of an unseemly Carriage' between Angus McDonald, a married man, and Isobel Campbell, who had previously been his servant. It was alleged that at a wedding the two had gone off together '& were afterwards found in the Cows Stalls in the Dark'. Not only that, but the following morning they were seen in the same bed, 'by which scandalous behaviour they gave great offence to every Serious Christian in the Neighbourhood'. The woman admitted going off with the man but insisted that she was not 'at any time off her feet but only Leaned with her Elbow upon the stall that was next the Door'. Asked what she was doing there with him, 'she could give no satisying account but at last said that she was Craving him… for her wages he was owing her and being further interrogate if or not her head Cloathes came off and if her hair that was taped up came down she says she knows not but the Plaid that was about her head and her hair might [have] come down.' As for the events of the following morning she said he only 'stretched himself upon her Bed but did not touch her'. Angus McDonald was called, and his story was that he had been in drink the night of the wedding and did not recall what had happened. He denied being in her bed the next morning, 'but being told she confessed it he acknowledges he did lay himself down in it he again & again prevaricated & could give no good reason for their being together at all.'

In the weeks that followed, various witnesses who had seen the couple together gave their evidence. By February the session decided that 'as the Parties seem to think but little of the Scandal because the actual guilt of uncleanness is not proven against them, that this whole affair should be referred to the presbytery.' It was subsequently reported that the two of them had travelled together to the meeting of presbytery and spent the night in the same bed in a lodging house, 'by which it would apear they were two impudent abandoned Creatures.' This case is unusual in that the couple were so brazen and as a result were punished as adulterers; but it does illustrate the attitude that one could resist accusations of fornication if not actually caught in the act or pregnant.

The Church strongly disapproved of physical contact or demonstration, and would regard it as scandalous carriage. In Longforgan in 1685 there was even a ruling that 'no Brydegroom kiss his Bryde before the minister' on pain of a fine of ten merks. Even two people of different sexes taking a walk together could lead to an investigation, the calling of witnesses, and even if nothing more could be proved, a reproof. The level of intimacy which, in an English church case, could be claimed as 'honest courtship' would, in Scotland, initiate a detailed enquiry.[3] Of course, the Kirk acted only when information of unseemly conduct was brought before the session. It is possible that practices such as night courting and bundling, known to have existed in the mid-nineteenth century, also existed in our period but were considered acceptable and not reported. It is, however, difficult to square the idea of such practices with the conspicuous evidence that Kirk and populace were in good accord on standards of personal conduct.

Another type of scandalous carriage occurred in Cramond (September 1707). Samuel Johnstoun was accused of unseemly behaviour with Agnes Bryce on the way home from Edinburgh. He declared that he and she, along with some others, drank a quart of ale, but that 'neither he nor she wer in drinke'.[4] 'Being desired to tell the truth whither there was any miscarriage between them by the way? he denyed, but said that she haveing a sore foot, satt down on the ground to looke it, & he satt down beside her, Being asked, If he kissed her & he answered, he did.' Two witnesses were called, and their versions went further than kissing. George Mure, a 60-year-old man, declared he saw the two of them at the highway side, 'and him between her leggs, and then he lifted up her cloathes & was Lying above her, he was not long above her, he pulled her up again & could not gett her kept up, she was so in drinke'. Mure's younger companion confirmed the story, adding that when he saw Johnston 'well up her coats, & Ly doun above her' he had caused Mure to call out to them in order to 'hinder them to committ sin'.

What was the dividing line between acceptable and unacceptable courtship practices? An illustrative case arose in Thurso (March 1722):

> Donald Manson Sailor & Christian Nicol formerly delated of scandalous behaviour viz of walking together at unseasonable hours and particularly their sitting together one night a little above the Chappel of pennyland betwixt the hours of ten & eleven at night and he the said Manson sitting hard by her with his arms about her neck,

both of them being cited... acknowledged what was delated against them to be truth... but at the same time they declare that the design of their meeting upon that night was to concert matters with respect to their contract & marriage and that they would not frequent one anothers company so much if they had not intended to marry very soon. The Session finding... that the foresaid Donald Manson sailor is in suit of her and that they actually Intend to marry and likewise considering that nothing can be proved against them but what may be allowable to persons that intend to marry do give up with this process.

In permitting behaviour that without that intent to marry would have been punishable, this session revealed exactly where it drew the line. Unfortunately, it is the only instance we found of a couple cited for scandalous behaviour who were let off any penalty because they were going to be married. Perhaps such couples tended not to be cited before sessions, since the sessions would already know of the marriage plans and make due allowance; we cannot know. What is clear, however, is that a practice such as 'bundling', or courtship in bed, accepted in certain peasant societies, was utterly opposed by the Church of Scotland. In Kilfinan, in December 1721, the kirk elders learned that Duncan McCurrie and Isobel Midy had shared a bed while working at the harvesting in the Lowlands. McCurrie was called before the session and stated 'That he lay in Naked bed with Isobel Midy the tyme of their being in Lothian at the shearing in harvest last, that it was the Custom of the place for Neighbours and Country bairns to ly together and that there were many others who lay together as they did: he absolutely denied any Carnal dealings with her.' She concurred and they were subsequently purged by oath of fornication. However, 'The Session Considering the baseness of the above practise of single persons bedding together, the offence given thereby to the Christian people and to be a warning to others for the future', they both had to make public appearances and be rebuked before the congregation.

Christian Barker of Wemyss (March 1755) was cited for indecent behaviour with a man who, she claimed, was courting her, and insisted that 'she would give over her Bed and sit by the fireside herself'. The session decided that 'her Excuse was only a sham and a shift' and ordered her to appear publicly. This woman already had a bad reputation for having strangers in her house, and the man was not known to the session. However, the fact that, barring the Thurso case above, none of the couples cited for scandalous carriage tried to claim courtship as a valid reason for their actions indicates that any kind of physical intimacy was considered unacceptable for an unmarried couple.

The absence of claims that marriage was promised has a direct bearing on the theory of 'failed courtship' in fornication cases. If the pregnant girls had expected their partners to marry them, then surely they would have said so, particularly if they girl had been abandoned or repudiated. In fact, this defence or excuse was not offered. Even the phrase 'under promise of marriage', which occurs in some places in the 1660s and 1670s, virtually disappears after that. In Wemyss, in January 1661, Geills Bred admitted fornication with David Beans, her servant, 'and being Inquired iff his filthines comitted was under promise of mariadge Answered negatively'. The man 'declaired he hade so often comitted the act of filthines with hir in hir own bed he could not give ane particular Accompt And being Inquired iff the samen was under purpose of mariadge Answered negative'. At a later date the question would not even have been asked. The word 'filthines' conveys the session's revulsion at

Girls in Trouble

unmarried sexual activity.

In one case a woman alleged pregnancy to get a man to marry her. In November 1741, Margaret Barbor of Rothesay claimed to be pregnant, but the man named as father denied guilt. The local community believed it was a pretended pregnancy, 'as a wheedle to noose him into marriage', and on 6 December the woman was examined by midwives who found no signs of pregnancy. It may be that a woman did think she stood a better chance of getting her partner to marry her if she were pregnant, but we do not believe from this one case (where the pregnancy was fictitious) that women would get pregnant for this purpose.

The low level of pre-marital pregnancy, as shown in Chapter 5, demonstrates that sex before marriage was rare. This leads us to dismiss those popular ideas that it was customary, at least for Scotland. One old chestnut is the supposed seigneurial right to intercourse with girls before or at their marriage, the so-called *jus primae noctis*, a theme associated with *La nozze di Figaro* and resurrected by *Braveheart*. The Kirk could not have failed to condemn such a practice, and the lairds who imposed it, but nowhere is it mentioned. One who claims it existed is Tom Johnston (in his *History of the Working Classes in Scotland*), but he bases this on statements by Boece, Buchanan, Skene and Boswell, who in turn relied either on hearsay or on each other. The right, or practice, was also suggested scurrilously by Thomas Kirke in 1679. These accounts place it far in the past, and so does the fictional description of it by George Mackay Brown. Frankly there is not a scrap of worthwhile evidence for the practice or the right to it, not only for Scotland in our period, but for any place or time in Christendom.[5]

If expectation of marriage was not the reason why many girls had sex, then why did they do so? Proximity, opportunity, and lust? A young man and a young woman serving together in the same household would be thrown together frequently, and the large proportion of cases involving fellow servants – echoing a trend found in England – shows that this temptation was hard to resist. The master and mistress of the household were supposed to keep an eye on their servants, but this was not always feasible, or not always carried out.

The world of our cases, for most of our period, was one of very limited material possessions. In Belhelvie, in January 1741, Elspet Davidson was pregnant by her fellow servant George Rheney. Their master told the session of malicious rumours that he had made them lie in one bed together, so he wanted them both to swear they slept in separate beds with enough bedclothes on each. They did swear but later claimed that he had bullied them into denying the truth, which was that on a very stormy night Rheney's bed had been too cold to sleep in and their mistress had told him to sleep in Elspet's, knowing full well what was likely to occur.

Close contact with fellow servants of the other sex was not supposed to happen in bed, but the working life of many girls gave ample opportunity for sex. In particular, the frequency with which girls were made pregnant by their master or their master's son shows how easy it was for someone with authority to create opportunities. Such liaisons were not necessarily coercive, as many young people were placed in households of roughly the same social status as their own, very often the houses of kin.

There were also couples who did not serve together, so where did they have sex? In most cases for which we have details, even in summer it happened indoors rather than outdoors. This is not surprising given the Scottish climate (though the same was also true in seventeenth-century Somerset[6]). It might be in the house where the girl was employed if she was in service, or her father's house if she was not; it could be the man's house, or the house of a friend or relative. There may have been connivance in some instances, but for the most part it seems that a couple simply took advantage of an empty building. In Dysart (May 1669), when Elspet Whyte was asked where James Martin had had carnal dealing with her, she 'Answered in William Cunygham's house being posed wher was the folkes that belonged to the house Answerd that William Cunyghame was not at home and sume body cryed to his wife to goe to the yeard and in that tyme he lay with hir.' Also in Dysart, in February 1760, William White, the man named as the father of her child by John Ramsay's servant, Margaret Pringle, admitted that 'on the Friday after Leslie Mercat he went into John Ramsay's house when he knew that neither he nor his wife were within on ane ill design.'

Aside from houses, other indoor venues were stables, barns, byres and mills. There are statements such as 'in his barn' and 'in his brother's byre'. These were places where servants sometimes slept and also places where the risk of discovery was small. Opportunities for intercourse were often seized during work. In at least one instance, that of Isabel Gardiner and William Suine in Dysart (October 1762), the two of them had been 'brewing in the Stable where his horse stood'. This apparently could go on until very late at night, for 'she affirmed That many times he had been with her at the brewing business till two or three a clock (in the morning).'

Another instance of a sexual encounter at work comes from Wemyss, November 1721. It was alleged by Beatrice Turnbull that, after the other workers left the workshop, Mr Orme, in charge of it, said 'Stay Beatrice, and I will give you the Receipt your father was speaking off for some iron. Then he shut the door, and strugled with her'.

Mr Orme waited till the two of them were alone, but privacy was not essential. It is difficult for people today to realise how rarely people in early modern society enjoyed privacy. Three to a bed was a common feature of life.[7] Intercourse could take place between a couple with a third person in the bed. (Of course, hard outdoor work might make the third person sleep heavily: certainly in several cases such people were found to be useless as witnesses.) In Dysart (August 1702), Margaret Simson 'acknowledged that she was frequently guilty of Adultery with the said Alexander Bans and that they were once guilty of it in Jannet Gordoun's House Janet Gordoun being in the bed with them in time of the action.' In Kilfinan (November 1744), John McLane denied Mary Smith's assertion that he had had intercourse with her at the Smith's house at the ferry of Otter, 'where the Landlord of the House Jo MacFarmling desired them to go to bed together.' Katharine Smith was called as witness but could not say whether intercourse had taken place, as 'after having lien down in Bed beside them [she] fell immediately a Sleep'. In Dysart (August 1767), Catharine Gilmour stated that 'when it was very late she & her Comerade went to bed, & that James came to bed to them a little after they had gone to bed – & then & there was guilty with her.' She subsequently added that 'James had been guilty with her both when her Comerade was in bed with her & asleep & also after she had got up in the morning she having got up before her & James.'[8] However, the presence of a third person in the bed was sometimes put forward as evidence that no misconduct could have taken place.

Outdoor work also provided many venues for intercourse, including, in Wemyss, 'at the water side of Leven', 'at the double dykes between Newtoun and

Brankstoun', and 'in the Middle of Weems Mure'. In the Western Highlands the act often took place 'in the mountains'. As in seventeenth-century Somerset, sex was often the result of outdoor employment.[9] Distance from other workers gave opportunity. Beatrix Spittle, in Wemyss (February 1714), was guilty with George Bairner 'in the fields at a place called the horsehill the time the corn was stowing when she went with him to see what corn should be stowed [cut]'. In Dysart (April 1776), Janet Graham was guilty 'on a tuesday in May last pretty late at night, at the foot of the Pipers Braes, when she was agoing to wash to Mrs John Brodie'. In Kilfinan (May 1755), in the Highlands, Isabel Mun stated that 'their first Carnall Dealings were att the Peat-Moss, att the time they were Leading home the peats.' Also in Kilfinan (November 1744), Betty Stewart stated that Archibald Lamont had been guilty with her 'about the 22d May between Kildair and Aird when she was thigging [acquiring] wood'. And in the same parish (October 1748) Dorothy McDonald claimed that Dugald McLauchlan 'had first guilt with her as they were attending some Cattle on the hills of Faylan'.

Travelling together to or from fairs or markets also provided temptation and opportunity. Helen Mackay (Kilmartin, February 1745) confessed guilt with Malcolm McBrian, smith, 'as they were both coming home from the first Foord Market upon a Friday'; which the session reckoned to be 27 July. Though the issue of drink was not raised in these cases, a visit to market could have included ale bibbing.

The season for outdoor sex ran from April to September. There was no seasonal pattern to indoor sex, which was far more usual. Special occasions, marriages or traditional saints' days (still observed in spite of Church disapproval), all gave opportunities for contact, for drinking and for staying in other people's houses, or, alternatively, might lead to the absence of those who might prevent love-making. In Dysart, in December 1669, Joanit Archibald was made pregnant in 'John Dalrumpil's maltbarn... upon that day which John Williamson was married.' In January 1775, Barbara Miller claimed the first offence was on 'the saturday evening before Kirkcaldie sacrament at the east side of James Horn's dyke', the second on 'the thursday before the king's birthday' and a later episode on 'the day of Gallowtown market'.

As Chapter 2 described, women were an essential part of the rural labour force, and it was quite common for a woman to work alone, or with only a man as companion, or to be sent on a distant errand alone. Housing was cramped, and if extra people arrived at a house they would share the beds already in use. Protection or chaperonage for women was impractical. More importantly, there was not a felt need for it in this period; the expectation was that both sexes would observe the moral codes unsupervised. This is very different from the ethos of the mid- or late-nineteenth century, when the upper classes strove to prevent servants having the opportunity for sexual encounters and when the respectable working class of the cities also endeavoured to protect and segregate the womenfolk.

There is little indication of disapproval of girls being in situations where there was a risk of vigorous seduction, though in May 1699 the session of Kells 'taking to their serious consideration the unnecessary and unseemly converse of some young women with strangers... on fairs and publick mercat days' ordered all young women 'to keep themselves at a distance from strangers and lascivious young men'. Note that the duty of separation was placed solely on the women; though the young men were labelled 'lascivious', there is no censure of them in the ruling.

Given the opportunist nature of many of the encounters that led to illegitimate births, one might expect the economic changes of the later eighteenth century to have produced a marked change in patterns of sexual behaviour. All Scotland, though to different degrees, was experiencing more frequent movement of people, accompanied by a desire for greater personal independence. In the Lowlands there was a trend towards larger units of work, bigger farms, and industry organised on a wider and more regular system: in many places there were larger units of settlement as towns expanded and planned villages were set up. But larger work forces on the farms led to the use of labourers rather than living-in servants, and the demand for well-muscled labour and the need for nimble-fingered textile workers tended to segregate the male and female workforce. There was also a marked increase in real incomes, and consequently more comfortable and better equipped houses. The box bed, which created internal divisions within rooms, was an important step towards some privacy, and the availability of more furniture and the creation of more inns both reduced the occasional need for bed-sharing between the unmarried of different sex. In the 1770s there is evidence of considerable unemployment and dislocation in the Lowlands, which may have frustrated some prospects of marriage.[10] Some of these various economic changes might be expected to enhance, and others to reduce, the opportunities for unplanned sexual intercourse. The absence of a trend in illegitimacy, except for the rise in Ayrshire and the south-west, suggests that the effects cancelled each other out.

Girls in early modern Scotland (like those in seventeenth-century Somerset[11]) usually claimed that they had been guilty with only one man and on only one or two occasions. That second claim is dubious, given the low probability of becoming pregnant from one or two acts of intercourse, but it does indicate that such behaviour was considered less reprehensible than frequent couplings. As the kirk session made no distinction in punishing a girl who had sex only once and one who had done so on a number of occasions but with the same man, the values being reflected were those of the community rather than the Church. A typical statement was made by Mary McNiel in Kilfinan (February 1751): 'it was about february 14th in Innins Barn in the Daytime and that they only had Carnal Dealings together once'. Likewise Beatrix Spittle, whom we have already encountered stowing corn, said that 'she was never guilty with him nor any other person before or since that time.' However, Isabel Mun, previously noted as having sinned the first time when leading home the peats, was not able to make the claim of once only. She was able to give a clear account of a second encounter, but then went on to say that 'as to the third time they had Dealings she Could not particularly Condescend upon. But that they met Several times which she Could not Call to memory.' Geills Bred and David Beans, quoted earlier, did not appear particularly ashamed of their behaviour, but Mary Livison (Kilfinan, November 1751) seemed aware of having compounded her sin. After giving a precise time and place of guilt with John Mun she was asked 'whither or not they met but that time – att this she paused, but att Last told they had frequent meetings in the month of January but not after that.'

Some women named more than one man as guilty with them at about the same time, which could lead to problems in establishing paternity. For example, in Blair Atholl, in August 1744, Ann Robertson alleged that Duncan Robertson was the father of her expected child. He admitted guilt in January 1745, when she also confessed that she had been guilty with Angus McDonald, and that McDonald was the real father. McDonald admitted guilt, but denied fatherhood. Altogether we found 28 cases of women who, when challenged to name their partner, admitted, either then or later, that they had been guilty with more than one man at roughly the same time. This must be seen as in a different category from the successive liaisons which led to repeating illegitimacy.

Any sexual encounter which was considered incestuous led to a much higher level of penalty. We discussed in Chapter 3 the Church's definition of incest, and looked at cases of marriages that were considered incestuous. Here we look at cases of fornication that were placed in that category.

The risk of an accusation of incest with its very high penalty could lead to belated attempts to conceal the link. In Dundonald (August 1787), Margaret Porter claimed to have been raped by a stranger in circumstances that the session rightly regarded with scepticism, 'considering how improbable this was that ane could find ane opportunity for ane rape in the day time in a road so frequented'. It turned out that the man involved was her brother-in-law. A typical description of the woman involved in a case is that in Kilwinning, January 1784, 'a sister daughter of his deceased wife'.

Incest also covered cases where, by the Church's standards, affinity had been established by sexual relationship without any marriage. For instance, in Dailly (August 1731) Mary McBroom was alleged to be pregnant to a man lodging with her and her sister also accused him of her own pregnancy. The case was referred to the presbytery as an allegation of 'horrid incest'. Similarly in Pencaitland (March 1656), a man was referred to the presbytery for having got Agnes Wedderburn with child and having behaved with scandalous carriage with her sister Jean. Jean was not pregnant so it was merely 'a great presumption of incest'. In August 1712, in Wemyss, by contrast, an old liaison with a man was considered to have created a relationship which caused fornication with his nephew to be incestuous: Katharine Henderson, a trilapse case, had committed fornication with the uncle of her first bastard.

These instances show how an 'incestuous' relationship could, in some cases, be the result of ignorance of one of the participants of the sexual activities of the other, and that most cases labelled incest were not the result of sexual activity within a common household. The absence of instances of incestuous relationships between near kin does not mean that the most likely forms of such incest, between brother and sister and between father and daughter, did not happen, but only that any procedure initiated by obvious pregnancy was unlikely to pick them up. That incest of near kin certainly existed is shown by a very murky case of brother and sister incest in landowning society, which took up the time of the synod of Glenelg in the 1740s.[12] Such incest of near kin occurs predominantly when the girl is young, and from what we know of physiological development in early modern society, is unlikely to have led to conception in girls under seventeen. Yet most young people left their parental home for service of one kind or another before that age; in Scotland usually between the ages of ten and fourteen. Sexual encounters with these juveniles would seldom involve pregnancy. They would belong with other types of sexual irregularity, for instance homosexual intercourse, child molestation and bestiality, recorded only when direct evidence of the activity was produced. One KSR mentions a man emerging from behind a horse looking decidedly flushed, but

6: Where, When and Why

there was insufficient evidence to bring a charge of bestiality. In Penninghame, August 1706, the schoolmaster was accused by two girls of having laid hands on their private parts when beating them. He cleared himself on oath, and the session decided that the accusation sprang from a mixture of malice and the desire to be free of school. But the allegation, in September 1721, against William Young, schoolmaster of Dunkeld, that he had lain with several girls aged between seven and thirteen, and even abused a four year old, was sustained. He admitted the charge and was imprisoned.[13] But such instances of sexual aberration are rare in the records, presumably because there was seldom enough evidence on which to pursue them.

We commented in the last chapter that we did not systematically record adultery by married women since the child would not legally be a bastard. Such cases normally came to light only if the husband was away, or if there was good evidence, as in Dysart (August 1671):

> William Huttone declared that his wife Annas Mathie lying in a roome above him, he wakened about 3 or 4 hours in the morning, & heard a noise above, upon which he arose and chapped at the door, & with difficultie won in... having got in, she would have had him first search the chamber, but being suspicious he raised up a feather bed lying on the floor, under which was John Corser, who desired him to hold his peace & he would give him a pynt of aill.

With married women whose husbands had deserted them, the session was not always certain whether to treat their subsequent liaisons as fornication or adultery. In some instances the woman's allegation that her husband must be dead was eventually accepted. In Foveran (May 1695), Margaret Shepherd was able to produce a paper signed by the commissary clerk of Edinburgh stating that the husband who had deserted her some fifteen years before was dead. By contrast, at Longside (December 1710) Christian Dalgarno's statement that her eleven year absent husband must be dead was not allowed to be more than a strong presumption, and the case was labelled adultery.

This was an age before death certificates, and death could be accepted without formal documentation. In February 1677 in Ayr, Marion Cunyngham's husband, who had deserted 12 years earlier was considered to have died because some seamen had stated before witnesses that he was dead. Similarly, in Golspie in March 1747, Jean Bain was relieved of the accusation of adultery by some witnesses stating that her husband had died at Fontenoy. In Dalkeith (January 1697), Jannet Wilson's allegation that her husband had died two years before in Flanders was not proved – and indeed the fact that she then fled the parish would suggest that the claim was spurious – but her partner was allowed to appear for fornication only.

Evidence of a spouse's death did not necessarily absolve the other from the guilt of adultery if it proved to be incorrect. In a case in the Court of Justiciary in 1673, a wife had arranged for a fraudulent testimonial of her death in Virginia to reach her husband, who married again on the strength of it. By nine to six the judges held him guilty of adultery but then pardoned him. It is doubtful that a church court, even in the seventeenth century, could have taken such a severe line.

Much more common was adultery between a married man and an unmarried woman. Unmarried female servants were in an unprotected position, though girls who consorted with married men were under no illusions that this could lead to marriage. As shown in Chapter 3, while divorce, both for adultery and desertion, was

Girls in Trouble

recognised by both Church and State in Scotland, in none of the several hundred rural cases covering adultery or desertion which we have seen was the possibility even mentioned (though, as can be seen in *Sin in the City,* it was resorted to by some city dwellers).

Apart from the attentions of upper class men to lower class women, most of our cases involved men and women of similar standing. One curiosity was the case of Sipio Kennedy in Kirkoswald (December 1727), described as 'ye Blackmore in Culvan'. The session asked the presbytery for advice as the man was not a member of the church, though the session believed he had been baptised by an episcopal minister. Following the presbytery's recommendation, the man swore that he adhered to the Christian faith, and he duly made his public appearances before the congregation. There is no hint of racial prejudice in the recording of this event.

In most cases the women were, or at least appeared to be, willing participants in the act of sexual intercourse, but the possibility of rape obviously did exist. Scots law had been unwilling to concern itself with this crime unless the victim was propertied and had actually been abducted. In the matter of evidence it expected the victim to have cried out, and to have lodged a legal claim of rape within 24 hours. Our cases showed that seduction could be a fairly rough affair without the girl calling it a rape. In Lochgoilhead (October 1752), Jean Luck said the man responsible for her pregnancy was William Hind or Hay, 'she did not exactly know which', a travelling packman who was lodging at a nearby alehouse. She had gone to the house on

> an Errand and saw him sitting at the fire with some Punch before him and that he gave her a glass upon some acquaintance she hade formerly with him at Lochgoilhead, and that she left them to goe home and that he followed her and caught her before she got home that she cried but his landlady's assistance came too late and found them only talking together at her father's door.

Cries notwithstanding, given the circumstances described, Jean Luck could hardly be classified as altogether unwilling.

It was not unusual for statements to include an allegation that some degree of physical roughness had been used.[14] It seems that roughness, in the eyes of the community, was a normal part of life: rape meant real violence. In February 1720 in Kilmarnock an unmarried pregnant woman, Janet Stevenson, alleged not only violence, but that the man had forced snuff, or something like it, up her nose, and 'disordered' her for many days. Two other cases of rape came from the Eastern Highlands. In Blair Atholl, August 1751, Christian McFarland had reported to her family that she had been raped, and her father had told her to keep quiet about it: it was the pregnancy that brought the story out. Here it seems that being raped was itself a cause of shame. In Croy, in November 1761, witnesses assured the session that Ann Sinclair had been raped, and the session's comment was that she was 'more to be pitied than blamed'.

One case of attempted rape is worth quoting at length (although it is not entirely clear how far the man actually went) because it presents such a vivid picture of horseplay between the sexes, including the words used by the participants. Anna Swannie complained to Canisbay session (August 1731) of James Groat's violent treatment of her. The main witness declared that on the day in question he had been pulling heather along with Groat and another man, Charles Banks, when they saw the woman and wondered who she was:

6: Where, When and Why

> Charles Banks wager'd half of his dinner with the Declerant that he would not take a kiss of her Whereupon the Declerant call'd to her, inform'd her of his wager & asked a kiss to which she reply'd it was not usual for a young Rogue to kiss an old wife like her That then he softly laid her down & took one or two kisses from her But meant no harm.

After some more idle chat the woman had left them, and

> was gone but a little way when James Groat said it was well Done to be with that Woman and Immediately pursued her That the Declerant called to her to take Care there was one following her when soon after they went out of his Sight who listening heard a Voice from the place he supposed they were Crying Murder murder That shortly after James Groat returning they asked him what meant he? What had he Done? To which he made a reply so horridly prophane that it Deserves to be Registrate no where but in Eternal Oblivion.

Although Groat denied guilt (i.e. penetration), the session, 'considering the odious nature of the sin itself, but especially the Dangerous Consequences which may ensue if it is not Exemplarly punish'd to the manifest hazard of Innocent Travellers whose Chastity is expose'd to the Insults of such heaven daring Villains', ordered him to appear publicly in sackcloth. The woman was not considered to have provoked the attack, and the idea that 'she asked for it' is totally absent from all our cases.

One other example of attempted rape should suffice to give the flavour of such cases. In St Ninians (December 1724), Isobel Key told the minister that on her way home the previous night Robert Moir had attacked her and had only been stopped from raping her by some others coming along. She testified before the session that Moir had

> let down his Breeches & discovered his nakedness to her, & damned himself but he would ly with her, calling her damned Bitch & Jade; & that when she was outfoughten, by good Providence, the said John Mitchel & some others coming the same road from Down to Keir, she got out of his hands to them, & he was hindred from committing the act.[15]

Apart from sheer male strength, there were other ways of getting sex under duress or without consent. For instance, men could take advantage of infirmity, mental or physical, in women. In some of these the woman was labelled 'ane Idiot' or 'almost an Idiot'. In Belhelvie (September 1721), Janet Simpson was described as 'known to be ane Idiot and deprived of reason from her Infancy'. For Elizabeth Stewart in Banff (April 1702), the fact that she was 'almost an idiot' did not prevent her being criticised for 'very bad fame' and recommended to the magistrate for deportation. The limited mental capacity of some women meant that it was difficult for the session to be sure that the sinfulness of the event had been truly registered and therefore repented. Margaret Gilmuire in Wemyss (September 1705) was described as 'grossly ignorant and altogether stupid and under no sense of her sin', and Jean Auchinleck in Dailly, who got into trouble twice, was described on the second occasion (October 1746) as 'brutishly ignorant'. Similar allegations of mental defect or ignorance in men involved in sexual offences are very rare.

Fornication by a minister or elder of the kirk session was particularly shocking. In

Girls in Trouble

Dysart (October 1673), even though the elder involved with Isobel Moyes was intending marriage, he was suspended from office indefinitely for fornication. In Wattin (December 1758), Kenneth Sutherland, an elder, got his servant Elspet Corner into trouble and resigned. In Rothesay, Janet Auld's case of November 1738 led to the removal from office of the ruling elder, Duncan Lea, which shows the session prepared to take on a man of relatively high rank. In April 1758, in Alves, the session was astonished when Thomas Laing, elder, stood up and confessed that he had got his servant, Isobel Naughty, with child and sent her away. The session recorded its amazement, since it had had no other word of the affair, 'and scarcely knew what to say to Thomas' whom it described as 'a poor wretched old man'. When it collected its thoughts on a subsequent occasion he was deposed.

The gentry class, from whom some of the elders were drawn, fell into rather a different category. The difficulties in bringing such men under their discipline are discussed in Chapter 7.

There are few cases of upper class women coming before the sessions. In Rothesay, Bethia Beith (July 1706) was the daughter of a minister, and she was sinning within her own class with the son of the lord provost of Rothesay. Similarly, Ann Beith, also in Rothesay (June 1709), the widow of a burgess, was in trouble with an ex-baillie. In Thurso (January 1710), Elizabeth Sinclair, daughter of a late laird of Barroustoun, was in trouble with another man of lairdly background, and in Kingarth Mrs Elizabeth Stewart (February 1693), also involved with a laird, was allowed to stay in her own seat during her public appearances.[16] We did not find any cases of women sinning with men of a lower social class.

A final question must be raised in this chapter, although our sources do not provide us with conclusive answers. How were girls who gave birth to illegitimate children in this period regarded; not by the Church, but by the community in which they lived?

In England the economic fears of an unmarried pregnant woman were strong, but she did not face the public shame almost inevitable in Scotland; her embarrassment would be confined to those living near or related to her. In our cases the economic plight was less severe than in England. As we shall see in Chapter 7, the Church coerced most of the fathers into admitting responsibility, and into contributing to the support of the child. If a woman could not gain help from her parents or her man, a parish would give some relief while she was nursing her child. We do not have comments about the willingness of masters to take on servants with children, but parishes assumed that once a child was weaned the mother did not need relief. In the first half of our period of study a woman moving to work in another parish would need to show a 'testificat' of conduct from her last parish of residence, and such a document would reveal her past, but if the sin was purged this would probably be no handicap to movement.

Malcolmson's study of English cases stresses the acute problems of a servant girl (for such the mothers almost always were) faced with pregnancy, loss of employment and inability to earn a living for lack of a character reference. The days of written references lay ahead, in the nineteenth century, though at English hiring fairs, farm employers would make enquiries about a worker's general reputation.[17] The picture given by Malcolmson seems to belong much more to the mid-nineteenth century, when most residential service in England – and Scotland – was for domestic work, and thus more intimate than farm work, and by which time the management of

6: Where, When and Why

household servants had become much more systematic. Thus, a major component of social control in the Victorian era, and one which remains powerful today, is control of personal conduct by employers and by the ethos of the workplace; but it does not seem to have been strong in our period.

For this reason, we should not assume that a girl's 'character' was permanently damaged by pregnancy, since most of the statements to this effect come from other countries or other periods.[18] As seen in Chapter 5, in the Eastern Highlands and elsewhere there were some cases of antenuptial pregnancy where the father of the child was not the husband, and where the husband does not appear to have rejected either the child or the wife.

There was, admittedly, a handful of cases where a woman complained that a slander was hindering her marriage. The first came before Petty kirk session in June 1765. William Sinclair was courting Jean McDonald when he met up with a previous suitor of hers, John McNicol, who told him that during the three years she had been a servant in his father's house she had 'made a practice of Bedding with him':

> The above narration of McNicols had such weight & credit with Sinklair that he declined agreement with this young Woman in Point of Marriage – But declined to give his Reason – being tender of the Girls Character – Till at Length being urg'd much to give in his Objections, he made plain all his mind as above.

The two men and the woman appeared before the session.

> Jean McDonald Complained of her being badly us'd by the affair & in order to Repair her Good Name begs of the Session to Take McNicols Oath whither or not he had ever committed Lewdness with her. She did not care to Require his oath if he had told Sinklair, or not, but if ever he was Guilty with her or not as no less would clear her of a bad Report.

The session agreed to this, and McNicol willingly swore 'That he had never any Carnal Dealings with the Girl either in the day time or nightime in his life.' The minister concluded by declaring to Sinclair 'that he had no Grounds of any further Objections against the Girl, and that now he might go forward in the intended Marriage when he pleased.'

Whether the marriage went ahead or not we do not know, but the above does act as an effective antidote to one particular notion that might have arisen from some of the material in this chapter. Chaperonage may have been lax and opportunities many, but there is a difference between attitudes in general and those of an individual toward a potential marriage partner.

Another piece of evidence comes from a book by David Stewart of Garth. Although written in the early nineteenth century, one gains the impression that the custom which he described was longstanding:

> For the illicit intercourse between the sexes, in an unmarried state there was no direct punishment beyond those established by the church; but, as usual among the Highlanders, custom supplied the defect, by establishing some marks of reprehension and infamy. Young unmarried women never wore any close head dress, but only the hair tied with bandages or some slight ornament. This continued till marriage, or till they attained a certain age; but if a young woman lost her virtue and character, then she was obliged to wear a cap, and never afterwards to appear

Girls in Trouble

with her hair uncovered, in the dress of virgin innocence.[19]

The custom of indicating that a woman was not a virgin is interesting because by accepted doctrine the unmarried mother had purged her offence. It was expressly stated in a letter signed 'A Country Elder' in the *Scots Magazine* for 1757 that penance re-established a girl's character, and that she could expect to marry later. The chances of subsequent marriage for those who had done penance are, unfortunately, not discernible from our material. But the view that character had been re-established was not simply a view of those managing Church affairs, as is shown by a surprised comment by Edmund Burt, writing in the 1720s, that 'When a Woman has undergone the Penance, with an Appearance of Repentance, she has wiped off the Scandal among all the godly, and a Female Servant in that regenerated State is as well received into one of the Families as if she had never given Proof of her Frailty.[20]

Notes

1. Much of the material of this chapter was published in the *Journal of Social History 22* (March 1988), pp. 483–97, under the title of 'Girls in Trouble: the social and geographical setting of illegitimacy in early modern Scotland'.
2. T.C. Smout, 'Aspects of sexual behaviour in nineteenth-century Scotland', in Peter Laslett, Karla Oosterveen and Richard M. Smith (eds.), *Bastardy and its Comparative History* (London, 1980), pp. 211–13.
3. M.J. Ingram, 'Church courts and neighbourhood: aspects of social control in Wiltshire, 1600–40' (unpublished D.Phil. thesis, Oxford University, 1976), suggests considerable tolerance of physical familiarity between the sexes in the early seventeenth century.
4. A Scots quart was two and two-thirds the size of an imperial quart.
5. T. Johnston, *The History of the Working Classes in Scotland* (Glasgow, 1922), pp. 12–13; Thomas Kirke, in P. Hume Brown (ed.), *Early Travellers in Scotland* (Edinburgh, 1891), p. 258; *Encyclopaedia Britannica* (Cambridge, 1911), xv, p. 593 *Jus primae noctis*.
6. G.R. Quaife, 'The Consenting Spinster in a Peasant Society: Aspects of Premarital Sex in "Puritan" Somerset 1645–1660', *Journal of Social History* xi (1977–8), p. 229.
7. It appears that there were gradations in status to different positions in the bed, the one nearest the wall being the most coveted position; cf. 'Captain Wedderburn's courtship', a ballad recorded by Jean Redpath, in which the man promises the woman the place in the bed by the wall. Presumably it was because the person on the outside would be the first one up, to unbar the door, stoke the fire, etc., and would have everyone else climbing over him or her.
8. The man claimed that he 'slept along with them all night – but that they had all their Clothes'. However, in July he finally admitted that the woman's story was true.
9. Quaife, 'The Consenting Spinster', p. 229.
10. Bernard Bailyn, *Voyagers to the West* (London, 1986), pp. 45, 198.
11. Quaife, 'The Consenting Spinster', pp. 232–3.
12. W. Ferguson, 'The problems of the Established Church in the Western Highlands and Islands in the Eighteenth Century', *Records of the Scottish Church History Society* xvii (1969–70), pp. 25–8.
13. Leah Leneman, *Living in Atholl, 1685–1785* (Edinburgh, 1986), p. 158.
14. Quaife, 'The Consenting Spinster', p. 240, 'Somewhat fewer than one in ten of the girls consented to sexual intercourse through fear or violence'.
15. For other attempted rape cases see: Longforgan, May 1718; Olrig, July 1723; Thurso, July

6: Where, When and Why

    1723; Belhelvie, August 1754.
16 'Mrs', i.e. 'Mistress', implied rank, not marital status.
17 Ann Kussmaul, *Servants in Husbandry in Early Modern England* (Cambridge, 1981), Ch. 4.
18 E.g. K.H. Connell, 'illegitimacy before the famine', in K.H. Connell (ed.), *Irish Peasant Society* (Oxford, 1968), pp. 55–62, claims that in nineteenth-century Ireland a mother of an illegitimate child had very poor marriage prospects; M. Ingram, 'The reform of popular culture? Sex and marriage in early modern England', in Barry Reay (ed.), *Popular Culture in Seventeenth-Century England* (London, 1985), pp. 129–65, states that a good reputation was of value for both sexes.
19 David Stewart of Garth, *Sketches of the Highlanders* (Edinburgh, 1822), vol. 1, p. 89.
20 *Scots Magazine,* August 1757; Edmund Burt, *Letters from the North of Scotland* (Edinburgh, 1974), I, p. 195.

7

Response to Authority

The majority of offenders admitted guilt and made their appearances before the congregation. Baptism would not normally be granted to an infant until both its parents had satisfied discipline, or at least provided surety that they would do so (not just for sexual misdemeanours but for Sabbath breaches and other offences as well). This was a powerful tool in the hands of kirk sessions, for though since the Reformation baptism was no longer a sacrament, the people still considered it very important.[1] In Thurso, in June 1737, the father of an illegitimate child whose mother had died in childbirth begged that the child be baptised as 'no Woman would engage to Nurse the said Child while unbaptised.' For parishioners it was important to conform to society's informal values as well as the formality of church discipline. In Foveran (August 1749) it was reported that Mary Hay had been put out of her mother's family and would not be allowed back until she had satisfied discipline; for this reason she was allowed to make just two appearances.

Kirk session registers do not record the feelings of those who appeared publicly before a congregation; however, wives' feelings were taken into consideration in two cases of married men who had sinned. The father of Katharine Gow's child (Wattin, February 1763) was Thomas Calder, a married man. The presbytery recommended that the session 'deal the more tenderly with him on account of his Wife Mrs Calder who is a Woman of a reputable, blameless Character'. In the second case (in Spott, November 1687) the man had got one girl pregnant before he married another. He asked if he could be rebuked privately 'because it will be A great grief to his wyfe if he should Appear in publict'.[2]

Although the degree of shame felt by individuals must have varied a good deal, yet some shame there must have been. Most accepted this, but some attempted to evade the consequences of their actions or defied the Church's discipline. It is this minority who form the subject of this chapter. Resistance to authority can tell us much about the functioning of that authority and about the society within which it operated.

We can divide our resistance into two categories, although naturally there is some overlap. The first part deals with behaviour which was not primarily a defiance of church rules, but rather a desire to avoid the consequences of bastard-bearing. Even without the threat of church discipline, an unmarried woman might deny being pregnant, flee the parish, attempt to abort the pregnancy, or abandon or kill the newborn infant while the men responsible might deny paternity. The second part involves members of both sexes who refused to conform to the rules of the Church.

It was not unusual for a woman called before a session to deny being pregnant, often perhaps because they were still trying to deny this calamity to themselves. Such women usually confessed a short time after. But Margaret Young (Kilmarnock, April

1693) continued to deny she was pregnant up to the day she gave birth.

An accusation of pregnancy was normally the result of visible swelling. However, Jean Hay (Belhelvie, January 1672) denied the charge and said it was 'a more dangerous sickness'; about a month later, poor lass, she died 'of a hydropsia', which explains the mistake.

Anything resembling morning sickness in a young woman could likewise provoke accusation. Jonat Chalmers (Drainie, June 1679) went so far as to bring a bill of slander against the woman who had falsely accused her of being with child. However, Isobel Hislop in Dalkeith, who denied being pregnant on 9 September 1737, claiming she was being treated for 'a trouble upon her body', was in childbed on 25 September. In Kinglassie (November 1710), Janet Christie was alleged to have brought forth a child. She said she had simply been ill. Her breasts were examined and no milk was found in them, so she was cleared.

The inspection of breasts by midwives was the objective test whereby a kirk session established whether a woman had recently given birth or was shortly to do so. In Kirkoswald (March 1767) the midwives who examined Margaret McTier's breasts produced the milk in a glass for the elders.[3] For many, the mere threat of a breast inspection was enough to make them confess. (To refuse to submit to inspection would have been taken to indicate guilt.) Others waited until the midwives found milk before confessing. And if a woman was innocent, by having her breasts inspected she could prove this.

It was, naturally, very much easier for a man to deny paternity than for a woman to deny pregnancy. Before scientific tests were invented, there was no certain way of proving that a particular man had fathered a child; nevertheless, kirk sessions tried very hard to pin down the man responsible for the pregnancy.

Men often denied guilt or paternity at the outset but within a comparatively short time would admit the truth of the accusation. It seemed to us worthwhile to quantify the cases in which the man named admitted fatherhood within a month of the allegation. It is a crude measure, for men might be out of the parish at the time of the allegation. But the percentages of speedy admissions showed some interesting features which suggest that as an index it is not meaningless. Table 7.1 gives the average levels of admission in the various regions.

The differences in level are striking. All the northern and highland regions saw 70 per cent or more admissions, the south-east and Central Lowlands stood near to 60 per cent, and the south-west and Ayrshire were well under 50 per cent.

By and large the level for each region was stable throughout the whole period. There was, however, a downward trend in the north-east, the Lothians, Fife and the central Lowlands. In the Western Highlands in the 1680s there was a dip below 30 per cent and in the south-west a strong downward trend from the 1730s which brought the figure to under 30 per cent by the 1770s. Clearly the men of the south-west were increasingly unwilling to stand by their women and support their illegitimate offspring, a pattern which is in sharp contrast to the rest of Scotland. Over most of the country in two out of three cases of child bearing outside wedlock a woman would not be left to support the child on her own.[4]

There were cases where a woman insisted that a particular man had got her pregnant but the man continued to deny it in spite of being cited before the presbytery. If there was no proof and the man did not yield to pressure there was little the kirk could do. Sometimes the man would come forward years later and

Girls in Trouble

Table 7.1: Admissions of paternity

Percentage of men, by region, admitting paternity within one month of being named

Region	Percentage
Lothians	62
Fife	61
Central Lowlands	60
Central and Eastern Highlands	70
Western Highlands	69
Aberdeenshire	75
North-east	78
Caithness	72
Ayrshire	46
South-west	42
National Sample	65

admit he was the father. For example, in Belhelvie Elspet Dickie's married partner denied guilt in June 1745 and confessed in January 1750. In New Abbey, when accused in December 1766, Sarah Douglas's partner refused either to confess or to deny and fled to England. He returned and confessed in June 1772. In Banff, Isabel Mackenzie's partner denied paternity in September 1764 and confessed to it in November 1774. KSRs do not reveal the motives for such belated confessions.

It was not unusual for a man to admit guilt but refuse to admit paternity until he saw that the date of birth corresponded with the occasion of fornication. If it did not then he might feel himself justified in denying responsibility. Margaret Farquhar's partner (Wattin, January 1733) denied responsibility for her child because it was born ten days too early, but the session considered ten days 'no matter of Debat' since it was common knowledge that he was the father. James Crawfoord denied being the father of Margaret Gow's child (Thurso, January 1740) because it was born fourteen days early. The process was laid before two 'gentlewomen', who declared that it was quite usual for a first child to be born twelve or fourteen days early. The session proclaimed the infant to be Crawfoord's.

As was seen in Chapter 5, sessions and society at large clung to the fallacy that the normal term of pregnancy was nine calendar months from the time of intercourse. The kirk sessions of Western Highland parishes were particularly obsessive about pinning down the exact date of fornication, and men were prone to deny paternity if the birth date was even slightly off their estimate. However, even in the Western Highlands this did not get them off the hook. Katrine Campbell's partner (Kilmartin, July 1749)

> demurr'd a little as to his being Father, and alledging in his defence that the birth of the said Child did not answer his time of guilt with her by the space of fourteen days. He was then told that as he had acknowledged guilt with her, he must be the Father of the Child, according to the Rules of this Church provided she was willing to clear herself upon Oath six weeks before and after the time of their guilt from having any carnal knowledge of all other Men.

7: Response to Authority

She did so and he caved in.

Sometimes the woman would shield her partner, especially if he was a married man, and the tale would then be told that she had been raped by a stranger. Elizabeth Scot (Foveran, August 1763) had enough imagination to describe a precise location: the unknown man had 'jumped out from a benty bush betwixt John Nicol's and the Black Dog'. Sessions were profoundly sceptical of all 'unknown man' stories,[5] for this was not a country where strangers roamed unnoticed or unchallenged.

Whether or not her partner admitted responsibility, the woman was still certain to bear the brunt of any penalty or shame. Obviously it was also far easier for a man to flee the parish and lose himself elsewhere than it was for a pregnant woman, although some women did try. This was easier in a border area like Dumfries and Galloway, where women frequently slipped over to England, or took ship for Ireland, to have their illegitimate babies. Simply fleeing to another Scottish parish was rarely a solution, since the elders there would insist on knowing who she was and what she was doing there. Even if she fled to Edinburgh ministers could track her down. Most of the women who fled appear to have done so in panic rather than by plan and often returned shortly after.

In Dysart, Fife, Elspet Still became pregnant by a married man, John Leith. She fled to Edinburgh, where she had the child. Then, after a letter from the minister reached Edinburgh, she fled again, this time to Montrose, where Leith's sister, Jean, gave the baby to another woman, on the pretext that its mother had died in childbirth. It was Jean who related this tale on 22 February 1691, but on 1 March Elspet returned to the parish, confessed, and submitted to church discipline.[6]

One woman who escaped altogether was Margaret Innes. On 24 July 1670 she fled from Aberdour (where she must have been in service) to her parents in Belhelvie, Aberdeenshire, where her father got her onto a ship to Holland. There is no record of her returning, and her father had to make public appearances before the congregation for aiding and abetting her.

Some women tried to abort the pregnancy.[7] It is impossible to quantify this because those who succeeded would not appear in the records, while the unsuccessful ones denied the attempt, and there was seldom any proof. Presumably women did not attempt abortion not just because they had no idea how to go about it but because there simply was no safe, reliable way to do so. The methods were a clumsy mixture of folk medicine and physical assault; we have not found any examples of instruments being inserted. It would be the belief that a certain method might work, rather than scientific knowledge, that motivated an abortion attempt. In Grange, in February 1732, Helen Graham claimed her partner had brought her pennyroyal and wormwood sage to make her part with child. In Dysart, Elizabeth Ogilvie (November 1756) alleged that her master was the father. Her mistress gave her the 'bitter apple' in a drink and made her lift heavy items of furniture. Elspet Cromertie (Canisbay, July 1751) asked to have a stone put on her back. Isobel Grig (Foveran, July 1679) was 'endeavouring to smoother and kill the child in her womb'.[8] Elspeth Jamison (Wemyss, September 1709) was 'indeavouring to put back the birth and for that end had been seeking the saving tree from the gardiners and did leap over the bastealie'. (Savin is a species of juniper said to have abortifacient properties.) Margaret Walker (Torphichen, September 1728) said her partner gave her herbs which she refused to take; also he had insisted he would deny being the father and she had said to him, 'God will not let you deny it.'[9]

In Mauchline, Ayrshire, Marion Anderson (January 1691) said she was given herbs to drink to abort the child in her womb by a woman who claimed to have got rid of hers the same way. In Wigtown attempts at abortion were made by three different women in the space of six years (September 1714, June 1718, and October 1720), which suggests some local 'wise woman' to whom girls would resort.

In Fossoway the same woman apparently attempted abortion on three separate occasions. On 21 June 1747, Margaret McCarter (also spelt McArthur) admitted fornication and named a married man who denied it. On 13 September she said she had 'parted with child' (miscarried) in mid-July and that the man had given her something which she took. In February 1755 she surfaces in the records again, witnesses alleging she was 'endeavouring to make away with the child in her womb'. The infant was in fact stillborn. On 2 May 1756 witnesses again alleged she was tampering with a pregnancy. She denied this, and the attempt failed, for on 11 May the beadle caught her trying to abandon her infant at the kirk door.

A woman sometimes carried a child to term without being noticed as pregnant and reported to the kirk session. This was a dangerous situation because then she might abandon or kill the child. Though child abandonment was never common in any parish it was higher between 1680 and 1720 than either earlier or later. A statute of 1690 laid down a presumption of murder on any woman concealing an unmarried pregnancy if the infant should die. This copied English legislation of earlier in the century,[10] but seems just to have codified existing practice.[11]

This law was assumed to apply only to the unmarried, though its wording was more general. A girl accused of infanticide had only to be convicted of concealing her pregnancy and not calling for help in labour to be considered guilty of infanticide, unless she could produce strong evidence to the contrary. The Church's attitude to concealment was severe. At Inveresk in 1710 a blind woman, Anne Davidson, was before the session for fornication, but when it discovered that she had not disclosed her pregnancy 'till she was delivered', the session sent the case to the presbytery, which passed it to the Lord Advocate. It ended with her receiving lesser excommunication and being referred to the sheriff. There is no suggestion that the child had not survived, and Anne Davidson eventually claimed that she had been irregularly married.

There are other cases of Church severity beyond the letter of the law. In April 1725 Christian Will, in Wemyss, was cited for concealment along with her mother, who must have known of the pregnancy since they shared a bed. They claimed that they thought her trouble 'a gravel' and did not call in outside help during childbirth: a neighbour's accidental visit was thought to have prevented child murder, yet clearly the woman had assistance from her mother during the birth. In Dysart, in October 1772, Margaret Spence gave birth in secret but it is not clear that the child died; in any case, the Solicitor General, looking at the evidence, refused to start a process. In Wemyss, in February 1707, Bessie Swine was afraid to tell her mother of the pregnancy and so had no outside woman with her during birth. In all these cases the offence appears to have been simply concealment, not the murder of a child.

In English courts early in the eighteenth century there was apparently a change in opinion among the men who made up juries. Any evidence of preparation for the birth, such as the collecting of scraps of linen, came to be allowed as evidence which would override the presumption of guilt.[12] But in Scotland severity continued longer, and seems to have gone even beyond the statute. In 1713 a girl who had told two people that she thought she was pregnant was convicted under the presumption, as was one in 1743 who had told the child's father under promise of secrecy. The nineteenth-century commentator David Hume felt that some of the judgments were 'slovenly', not justified by rigorous standards of proof, and that, in particular, the courts had heard several cases at a time, a process unlikely to lead to care and discrimination.[13]

In March 1740, Margaret Jameson (Ellon) had denied giving birth but examination of her breasts convinced the session that this was untrue. She then claimed to have miscarried at sixteen weeks and to have thrown the body in a pool. The elders went with her and found it. It was stated by the midwives to be perfect, and she was sent to the prison in Aberdeen. A similar case in Dysart (February 1729), where Margaret Spence admitted throwing a female child down a well without checking whether it was alive or dead, also led to imprisonment. She later changed her story and claimed it had been born dead. Anne Dempster (Kingsbarns, June 1750) persisted in denying having given birth even after milk was found in her breasts, but three months later the body was found and 'laid beside her in the prison'.

We do not know the end of all these stories. Grizzel MackGuffach (Fordyce, August 1746) claimed that her child had been born dead when its body was found buried in a cellar. Similarly, Agnes Mitchel (Torphichen, November 1737), who threw her child in a coal pit, claimed it had miscarried, but midwives said it was a full-term body. Janet Vaitch (Pencaitland, January 1691), who claimed that she 'saw a beast carrieing away the head' of her foetus which she had put in a hole, clearly did not convince the session that the child had miscarried. Registers do not reveal the outcome of such enquiries, probably because the cases passed into secular jurisdiction. KSRs were kept to record the Church's share in business, not to satisfy the historian's curiosity.

The last execution under the statute was that of Anne McKie in 1776: after that, though the law continued to be stringently operated, the prosecution settled for banishment. In 1809 the change in legal opinion produced a statute modifying the law: concealment was still criminal, but the sentence was only two years' imprisonment, marking the view that it was neglect, not evidence of murder.[14]

The Church concentrated on the fact of concealment, which could be regarded as a repudiation of its discipline. In Drainie, in January 1674, Christian Millan, who did not call for assistance at the birth and was suspected of infanticide, was merely made to stand in sackcloth, and in New Abbey, February 1766, Mary Turner, who claimed she had had assistance, was referred to the presbytery.

A girl might deny her pregnancy before society at large, or conceal it; but what did she herself believe was happening to her body? No one could have grown up in the countryside of that time, with its lack of household privacy and routine coupling of farmyard beasts, without some exposure to sex. But the Kirk discouraged explicit sexual conversation, so observation may not have led to knowledge. Even in the much more sexually explicit and articulated world of today, and with sex education in schools, girls can fail to know how their bodies change and why. And from biological knowledge to understanding and acceptance is a long step. We cannot agree with the legal opinion of the seventeenth and early eighteenth century that failure to disclose pregnancy was always a deliberate decision, made with intent to defy the law and society.

There are somewhat better grounds for the legal view that infant death in cases of concealed unmarried pregnancy was likely to be infanticide.[15] We should still recognise, however (as the law did not) that some concealed pregnancies led to stillbirths or to natural perinatal deaths.

The parishes we studied produced a total of only twenty cases of either concealment of pregnancy or infanticide, and in two of the concealment cases no action was taken. The eighteen cases where murder was alleged form just 0.2 per cent of our illegitimacy total. If we add to this the near 1 per cent of abandoned illegitimate children, foundlings, the number of women determined to get rid of their child is low, and much lower than English estimates. There were various statements in the Scottish press of the time which claimed that infanticide was unusually common in Scotland.[16] These were simply based on impression, and are not sustained by criminal or other statistics. Indeed, our figures suggest the opposite. The figures put forward for England are so much higher than those found in this study that, even if some infant bodies had been successfully concealed – and the wilds of Scotland give some scope for this – we still have to accept a far lower level of child murder in Scotland.

Among 8,429 instances of illegitimacy we found 78 cases of abandoned children, mostly in the late seventeenth and early eighteenth century. None were recorded for the Western Highlands and only four for the Central and Eastern Highlands. There were eleven in both the north-east and in Aberdeenshire. The highest figure was for the Lothians where nineteen were mentioned.

An infant could be abandoned either with the intention of having it discovered,[17] or with at least a willingness to let it die, but these were only possible if the pregnancy had indeed been concealed. With the collusion of others, some girls would have gone to the nearest town to deliver and abandon the child there. If it happened to be winter, as with the one left in Cramond in January 1688, no wonder the infant perished. One abandoned in the same parish in November 1733 was in such bad shape that the family it was boarded with by the parish insisted on a specially generous fee: however, it survived to enter apprenticeship at the appropriate age.

In Cramond, Dalkeith and Dysart foundlings were sufficiently numerous for the parishes at times to have more than one being supported. Ayr also had four in the period between 1661 and 1690, but as a town it might have been the place of deposit by rural mothers. Grange in the north-east had two foundlings to support in the 1720s, so had Eddleston in the Borders. But in most places they were so rare that registers would simply refer to support for 'the foundling'.

Not all abandoned children came from impecunious women. In September 1766, in Ellon, a newborn girl was put down outside the manse with an anonymous letter to the minister and elders and a 20 shilling note. The letter promised more money from time to time and requested that the child be baptised. But the child was not well provided for, apart from money, for the women who nursed and reared it had to be paid immediately to get a blanket for it. The interest of this case is that the abandoning parent could write; perhaps it was the father who left the child. In Torphichen, in September 1702, the session established that the child laid down in the parish a year earlier belonged to the daughter of 'the Lady Pottishaw'. The lady had to take the child back and reimburse the session its expenses in maintaining the foundling. In Yester, in 1668, a small local landowner was concerned that a foundling might be attributed to his wife and asked for a testimonial that she had recently been seen in good health.

Kirk sessions, faced with a foundling, were very concerned to trace the mother, both to satisfy church discipline and to avoid expense. The parish had to recompense the woman who nursed it. Once the child was weaned it was usually handed over to an elderly woman already on relief with some small extra monthly allowance and occasional funds for clothes. The parish would also pay school fees until the child could read and was conversant with the Bible. Support usually stopped at about age ten to fourteen, when the child would go into service. However, a parish might resume care, giving support and medical aid, if an apprenticed foundling fell ill, or material help if he was neglected by his employer. The same system was used for the care of destitute orphans, and both types of children would eventually grow up in the poorer part of the labouring classes. But some sessions took a less generous approach. During the famine of the late seventeenth century the session of Perth decreed (May 1700) that a girl foundling of five years was old enough to beg for her living, and stopped supply.[18]

Happy was the session that could demonstrate that a foundling was the responsibility of another parish. In November 1670, in Dalkeith, Margaret Thomson admitted abandoning her child there because it was the parish of the father, who had refused to accept paternity, driven her away with threats, and then fled himself. In April 1749, Janet McAlester in Kenmore left the parish before the birth of her child. Some years later the minister of Kirkintilloch was in a position to point out that the child, abandoned, had been supported by his parish. In 1758, Daviot parish in the Eastern Highlands spent one pound and six shillings tracing the mother of an abandoned child. There was the woman of Fossoway caught in the act of leaving her child. In 1772, the parishes of Dysart and Kennoway took legal opinion as to whether, in the case of a child abandoned in Dysart whose mother had been identified but not found, it could be proved that the mother belonged to Kennoway. St Ninians, in 1729, knew that its parishioner Agnes Dobie had laid down her bairn at a door in Linlithgow, and Forglen, in 1722, knew that Christian Reid had fled the parish, abandoning her child in Turriff. In 1707 Cramond was so certain that the mother of a foundling belonged elsewhere that it persuaded the presbytery to organise a search and located her a month later in Linlithgow. In most of these cases we do not know what clues were followed in the detective work. But a common ploy when an abandoned infant was found was one noted earlier in this chapter: to have a midwife examine the breasts of all unmarried women in the parish for signs of recent childbirth.[19]

So far, the cases considered have been ones where the main motive was the fear of penalty, formal or informal, rather than outright rule-breaking. But there were also members of both sexes who deliberately defied the rules of the Church.

As seen in Chapter 1, church discipline was never meant to be purely punitive. Offenders were supposed to understand the nature of their sin and truly repent. If they did not, sessions sometimes refused to absolve them though they had completed their public appearances. Sometimes a session would criticise a woman as too stupid to understand her offence and so not capable of penance. More rarely was a man so described. In Dalkeith, March 1670, Robert Liviston confessed to fornication but 'being very stupid and insensible of his sin' the session ordained him to be put in prison 'till he give surtie for his satisfaction and penance'.

A disability which impeded interrogation was being dumb. But Elspeth Robertson in Blair Atholl (January 1747) was able to communicate by pointing to the man and making signs, and Mary Laing in Ellon (May 1757) did the same with the aid of her mother-in-law (a term which in the eighteenth century described a stepmother). There were also linguistic problems in some areas. Janet Sinclair, in Canisbay, October 1726, did not understand English, which meant that the minister could not 'deal effectually with her conscience'; and in Alves, February 1762, the session decided not to cite a woman who 'neither speaks nor understands English'.

More serious was the issue of whether penitence was real. In February 1768, the session of Kinglassie refused to absolve Margaret Morton, a relapse, because she showed 'no sense of Shame in her Sin and particularly that she had been expressing Passion and resentment at the rebuke and no Sorrow for her repeated Scandal.' Attitude was all-important, and there must have been at least some hypocrisy by certain guilty parties. Those unwilling to humble themselves before the session suffered for it.

In Torphichen, a man and his wife were guilty of antenuptial fornication and it was a relapse, as the woman had already borne him a child. The elders reported to the session that

> they conferred with Archibald Glen & his wife; And that the said Archibald took it in good part; but that his wife being told by William Nimmo that her last fall with her husband before marriage was a sin; she commanded him to be silent, and he having enquired, whither she bid him hold his peace, for any fault of his own, or because he was commisionat by the session? she replyed. There had been over much of that allready, and Therefore he would doe well to be silent, else there would be worse of it.

The session considered her carriage 'most offensive and Insolent'. This occurred in 1704, and the session pursued the couple for years afterward; in 1707 they were referred to the presbytery, and not until 1708 were they considered sensible of their sin and absolved.

An unusually detailed description of a woman's involuntary response and the session's reaction appears in Forgandenny session minutes in April 1743. Margaret Anderson had been found guilty of incest, and the punishment decreed for her was that she must stand in sackcloth outside the church door between the ringing of the second and third bells. The session called her in and told her of this,

> But in intimating this their sentence as Shee was humbled in Sackcloth she uttered the following Words Namely oh I cannot stand there to make a Fool of myself upon which she was immediately removed and therupon the Session, being deeply wounded and exceedingly grieved at such an Expression she had dropt as savouring rank of a proud & unhumbled Heart & Spirit, resolved to delay taking her upon her publick Appearances till such time as they had ground to believe shee had such a sense of her sin as to deserve all the Punishment which they at least had thought proper to inflict on her Body, and to acquaint the Presbytery of this her insolent Behaviour.

She was called in and

> informed what great offence by such an Expression she had given to this Session Upon which she wept most bitterly and declared that what she meant by such an

Expression was That being very weak of Body at the Times she would not be able to stand so long without falling down and thereby would make a Fool of her Self but did not think the Session was dealing too harshly with her and did not in the least intend to give them any Offence.

The following week the minister reported that the woman had expressed her sorrow to him for offending the session and her willingness to do as they ordered. For his part, the minister, 'tho' he was very much stunned at the time of her dropping the Expression which had offended them he was now satisfied she did not intend thereby to offend them or show a Contempt of their Sentence.' The session was still determined to refer her to presbytery, but a week later an elder who spoke with her reported that 'he was really of Opinion shee was acting a sincere Part for that amongst severall Expressions she had in their Conversation together he could not but remark this one, which she uttered with a great Deal of Concern, Namely That if it would please the Lord to forgive her her sin shee would never forgive herself.' The session decided not to consult presbytery after all. There was a postscript to this case in October of the same year:

> It was represented to the session that Margaret Anderson was complaining that she was not able to stand without at the porch door betwixt the ringing of the 2d and 3rd Bells as heretofore she usually had done for most of the Sabbaths she had compeared by reason of the coldness of the weather The Session agreed to ease her of this Appearance without at the porch door as taking no Pleasure in the punishment of her body further [than] that as a Mean it might be blessed of the Lord for afflicting her Soul.

It was also Forgandenny session (May 1743) which resolved not to allow fornicators to continue public appearances unless they seemed humbled for their sin, 'because it was but too evident that the most part who were left of God to comitt such sins lookt upon their publick Appearances as a kind of Satisfaction & Atonement for their Crimes and thereby perverted the very Nature & Design of them as being only a Mean to bring them to a sense of and shame for their sins.'[20]

The most usual form of defiance of the Church's rules was a refusal to appear publicly before the congregation. Men did this far more often than women, but women also refused.[21] Sometimes the session prevailed on them to change their minds; those who proved incorrigible were deprived of church privileges, and a sentence of lesser excommunication was pronounced against them (the sentence of greater excommunication was rare). Often, some years later, an excommunicated man or woman would ask to have the sentence lifted, after agreeing to undergo the discipline decreed by the session. With so many important community rituals and events tied in with the Church, exclusion must have been a very real deprivation.

We did, however, find one whole community which defied the Church for some years. The salt industry was important along the Fife coast, and the kirk session of Dysart waged a longstanding battle to stop the salters profaning the sabbath by working their pans on Sundays.[22] In May 1745 a salter, guilty of antenuptial fornication, craved baptism for his child. The session minutes recorded that 'for some years past the salters have been denied Church priviledges by reason of working their pans upon the Sabbath day', but that this 'scandalous practise being now left off by them', the man was admitted to church privileges.

The language used about women who did not conform was strong. Janet Sinclair (Banff, June 1725) was 'a vile abandoned prostitute'; Janet Aberdeen (Ellon, March 1738) was 'reported to be a Strumpet'; Janet Strouk (Dundee, September 1743) was 'a notorious common Prostitute'; Margaret McIntosh (Croy, June 1760) was 'an old practitioner in wickedness'. In March 1714, the minister of St Ninians discovered that the testificat presented by Margaret Frazer was forged. He wrote to the minister of Kilwinning, the parish where she came from, who informed him that the woman was 'a great whore'. Whether these women were really prostitutes is unclear. The larger Scottish towns in the eighteenth century certainly had women who regularly sold sex, but words like 'whore' are often used in male descriptions of female sexual deviance.

In the rare cases of women whom a kirk session considered to be beyond redemption, recourse could be had to the secular courts. In February 1701, Rothesay session referred Anna McTimus, a relapse case, to the sheriff depute, who intended to keep her imprisoned and to have her head shaved in the public mercat (i.e. market) place. In Ayr in the 1770s, prostitutes were passed to the council which would exile them and scourge them. In Caithness, the sessions themselves ordered physical sanctions, which the town officials would carry out without any secular judicial process. In March 1716, Christian Machugh, a trilapse case, was ordered by Wattin kirk session to be put in the 'jougs' (i.e. an iron collar) for half an hour before service, and later was ducked, shaved and exiled. Thurso kirk session also used the 'jougs' for several sabbaths on Jannet McKinla in October 1716 for 'notorious prophaneness'. In December 1701 Barbara McKean was to be 'convoyed from the pit by the executioner with a paper hat on her head to the stool, her head to be shaven by the hand of the hangman'. After that she was to be thrown out of town by the hangman and promised a ducking if she appeared again. In Wattin, in October 1704, Jean Gunn was called 'a vile person unworthie of entertainment in a Christian society' and handed to the baillie for corporal punishment; and in Thurso, in March 1705 and April 1709, Elspeth Murray and Mary Sinclair were handed over to the magistrate for corporal punishment. What was expected was made explicit in October 1724 over Jannet Barrie: the magistrate was recommended to 'scourge her out of town' as a lewd woman.

So far we have dealt almost entirely with women, yet it was men who most consistently resisted the Church's authority, especially 'gentle' men. Promiscuity among men was not labelled as it was for women. In 1649 the synod of Lothian and Tweeddale was handling the case of a man guilty of 'septilapse' in fornication, but made no particular criticism of him.[23] Similarly, when a man was involved in more than one unmarried pregnancy at the same time, this would lead to no special comment. But even if sessions were not openly denunciatory, they would wear down refusal to acknowledge their authority, and in the end achieve apologetic or evasive replies. In Kenmore, in December 1752, Archibald Campbell, named as father of Cathrine McNucador's illegitimate child, acknowledged 'that he said to Anne Dewar. his former partie, when she was urging him to marrie her, That said Cathrine... and half a Dozen more girls were with Child to him at the same time; he was gravilie rebuked for thus scandalizing himself and others, and for making so light of the sin of uncleanness.' Campbell claimed that his remarks about Cathrine were 'a Joke to try what his Mother would say'.

We have discussed the connection between the gentry and the changing attitudes

7: Response to Authority

of the Church in Chapter 2. A particular difficulty faced by kirk sessions was to bring landowners under their discipline.

Caithness was an area of many small lairds, who were responsible for many pregnancies. In particular, the Kirk was frequently vexed by a group of families combining financial with sexual irregularity, the Sinclairs of Mey, Rattar, Murkle and the Earls of Caithness (minor members of the aristocracy whose landed wealth was small). The 9th Earl was a notorious reprobate and did not submit to church discipline. In Thurso, in December 1712, it was recorded: 'the session considering the Earls frequent falls into fornication, and that he has not as yet given any satisfaction, and is still contumacious, recommend it to the minister to advise with the Earl anent his case.' (Needless to say, the minister got nowhere.) There was also George Sinclair of Forss who displayed the same mixture: in 1728 his younger brother was advising him to find an heiress as a wife as a means of escaping from debt, but he never married and in 1729 he was delated for relapse in fornication.[24] In Canisbay (March 1735) Sir James Sinclair of Mey was 'admonished to avoid the Company of Base Women which besides the Sin and Guilt would reflect Dishonour upon him.'

Elsewhere, in 1719 and 1720, Alexander Robertson of Webster Straloch got three different girls pregnant without ever appearing before the session. In Rothesay kirk session register (May 1693) Issabel Austine named as father of her child the laird of Kaimes. Certain elders were ordered to speak to the laird 'discreetly and meekly'. The laird did in fact admit paternity in a letter craving baptism for the infant. He promised to make the requisite public appearances but did not do so. This is not atypical: in many cases it was clearly not a desire to avoid responsibility for the child which motivated these gentlemen, but rather the wish to avoid publicly humiliating themselves before men of lower rank. In Ratho (July 1698), Christian Goodale named as father of her child Alexander Foulis, laird of Ratho, and she was given 12 pounds for a quarter year's maintenance of the child; but when two elders called on Ratho he refused to meet them, saying, 'I have nothing to do with you'. In Dumfries, in July 1701, James Murray of Conheath denied being father to Bessie Maxwell's child, and continued denying it as late as 1706, although she said he had maintained it for the first three years of its life.[25] In Dalkeith, Anne Taylor named the Earl of Aboyne (July 1723), and said he had taken the child from her and 'sent it to the Nursing'. There is no record of the Earl's ever appearing before the session.

In December 1692, Cramond kirk session received a letter from Sir William Paterson of Granton saying that his gardener had begot a child with his servant maid, and asked to have the child baptised. The gardener submitted to church discipline although the woman fled. Such a case is, however, unusual; more typically the household of a gentleman who did not himself submit to church discipline tended to feel they could behave similarly. The difficulty which the kirk session of Wemyss had with the Earl of Wemyss and his staff over the years illustrates this point vividly.

In July 1706 Anna Thomson named the 4th Earl of Wemyss as the father of her child; he denied this. During the previous autumn she had been cited several times for having been alone with 'the Black who serves the Earl of Wemyss', although she had continually denied this. The session did not believe the Earl was guilty with her and rebuked her for 'scandalizing a person of his Lordships quality'. Paternity was never established. In December 1711 Anna Thomson was pregnant again; on this occasion the alleged father was the Earl of Wemyss's factor.

117

Girls in Trouble

In December 1713, Elspeth Simmers named the same Earl of Wemyss. The session asked her 'what evidence could she give to prove the same, for would any believe that a person of his quality, sense and education would be guilty of uncleanness with her a common coalbearer?', which seems rather naive on the part of the session. Her reply was that a number of people were aware 'that she was familiar with my Lord'.

The alleged father of Margaret Middleton's child (already born) was John Gordon, 'accomptant' to the 5th Earl of Wemyss. On 27 February 1729 it was reported that they 'had been suspected of living in a criminal correspondence together; but nothing ever could be found, as a Just ground of procedure against them'. On 9 April it was reported that she had confessed to the minister of Burntisland. Bringing her up the coast from Burntisland to Wemyss caused difficulties because her father would not put up bail and the Earl of Wemyss refused to concern himself in any way. Finally, by mid-April the session had Margaret in Wemyss, but was worried about keeping her as she had already made one attempt to escape. It was decided that the prison was too near John Gordon's house to be safe, and the session prevailed on Baillie Brown to keep her for just one night. That night Gordon started a 'tumultuous Riot at midnight having come with a partie, to have carried off the woman in a violent manner; but was happily prevented, taken prisoner and thereafter sent to Kirkcaldy prison'. Margaret Middleton was also imprisoned but later escaped.

Aside from the echoes of a more lawless age, these stories show how difficult it was for a kirk session to impose discipline if the local landowner did not support it. And, as a postscript, the Earl's next 'accomptant', Mr Adolphus Hay, was named as the father of Margaret Ross's child in July 1735. He at least did appear before the session and admitted guilt with her, 'but said he, I must look about me before I own the child.'[26]

We found in one session register the transcript of a letter which a pregnant girl, Margaret Smith, received from a young gentleman, Benjamin Forbes, 'son to Edinglassie' (Foveran, October 1748). As an expression of confused feelings of affection, dismay, moral obligation and self-implication on the part of a member of the gentry class, it could hardly be bettered:

> Margt I received a Note from you concerning your being with Child, which I'm sorry for, however your best is to leave the Town and go up the Country among your Acquaintances, for my Mother will be unsupportable if she find you out to be with Child in her Service. Since you lay the Blame on me, I can't help it, but since you do, if you have a Boy you'll call his Name Findlay. I'm just going to sail, so you'll best take my Advice and leave the Town.
> I am,
> Your Friend Benjamin Forbes
> P.S. If the child be mine it's been gotten when asleep, however, when I return to the country shall find the Certainty of that, and take Care of it, if it be mine. Adieu.

Benjamin clearly feared his mother more than he feared the session.

Once initial wrath had abated, it is likely that the Forbes family would have provided some sort of aid to Margaret. Others remained hostile, and with powerful legal and social weapons at their disposal. In 1712, a Selkirkshire woman wished to write to the mother of her lover, but was illiterate. She obtained help from William

Pringle, a Selkirk tobacco spinner, who wrote to Lady Broadmeadows at her dictation:

> Madam this is to lett you know thatt this child thatt I am with is to your son and none els. Madam I am very, sorry thatt such a thing should have been butt if you should have been never so angry it is worstt is myne and nott his for if I was going to Death I never a man in the world butt him So he needs nott take it to denayell for their is non the father of this child but him. This is from Betie Jenkison.

The family had Pringle jailed for two weeks and fined 12 pounds Scots for a criminal libel.[27]

As Chapter 2 showed, the landed in the eighteenth century could exercise a high degree of control over their tenantry, and legal decisions in 1750–1 made it very difficult for a parish to quarrel with a laird in the courts.[28] A landowner who belonged to the established Church might be an elder, and would in that case usually represent the parish in the higher courts. Yet kirk sessions, whether graced with a landowner's membership or not, were driven by moral not material values, and had in practice more effective authority over the mass of the people than had the landowners.

Some historians consider that the Church experienced a decline in power during the eighteenth century. In formal terms this was so, but so long as the mass of the population assented to Calvinist theology and the particular Scottish interpretation of it, the Church remained the dominant influence on society. We have indicated the ways in which some offenders attempted to evade penance and responsibility. This was almost impossible for women, and perhaps not surprisingly our material shows very few examples. For men the denial of guilt would not restore to them a clean reputation unless they were prepared to go on oath: by refusing to take an oath they could avoid financial responsibility. What is to us the most striking feature of our research is that over two-thirds of the men, in spite of some initial resistance in many cases, accepted discipline and responsibility. The Church, by its authority, was able to go a long way towards equality of treatment of the two sexes.

Notes

1 It was normal only for a man to present a child for baptism, but we did find Kilmarnock session allowing some women to present bastard children themselves.
2 The elders consented to this, though the minister was unhappy about it because it seemed to him unfair that the woman, who had been if anything less to blame than the man, had to make public appearances. As a compromise the session imposed a hefty fine on the man and announced this to the congregation.
3 An unusual feature of this case was that the milk was not considered proof of pregnancy. She had had a child about three years earlier and presumably went on breastfeeding for rather a long time.
4 A minor point of interest is that in Westerkirk, the parish with consistently higher illegitimacy than elsewhere in the south-west region, 60 per cent of the men acknowledged paternity.
5 For instance, Elspet Beak (Cramond, October 1673) was told that her story of a man, now fugitive, forcing her in the high street was 'most improbable lyke'.

Girls in Trouble

6   When the session first cited Elspet 'John Leith did draw his sword, and offered violence to two of the elders, who were sent to bring her to the session.'
7   There is no evidence of any form of contraception in kirk session material.
8   A. Macfarlane, 'Illegitimacy and illegitimates in English history', in Peter Laslett, Karla Oosterveen and Richard M. Smith (eds.), *Bastardy and its Comparative History* (London, 1980), p. 77, refers to the practice of tying the waist very tightly as a means of aborting the foetus.
9   He did initially deny guilt and paternity but admitted it a short time later.
10 Sir John Lauder of Fountainhall, *Historical Notices* (Bannatyne Club, Edinburgh, 1848), vol. 1, p. 224.
11 Mackenzie stated in 1678 that 'the Law presumes so far, a woman who has born a bastard, and has conceal'd her being with child, to be guilty of Paricide, if the child be found dead.' Sir George Mackenzie, *Laws and Customs of Scotland* (Edinburgh, 1678), p. 156. The Act is in *APS* ix 195.
12 In Surrey, where there had been cases of infanticide every 18 months, in only one case after 1727 was there a conviction; with the failure of severity, prosecutions fell off. J.M. Beattie, *Crime and the Law in England, 1669–1800* (Oxford, 1986), pp. 113–24.
13 David Hume, *Commentaries on the Laws of Scotland respecting Crimes* (Edinburgh, 1986), pp. 292–9.
14 The modifying statute is 49 Geo. III c. 14. For late cases under the 1690 Act, see John Burnett, *A Treatise on Various Branches of the Criminal Law of Scotland* (Edinburgh, 1811), pp. 571–5.
15 Keith Wrightson, 'Infanticide in early seventeenth-century England', *Local Population Studies* no. 15, (1975), pp. 10–12. Based on a study of Essex cases, he estimated that infanticide then ran at the level of 2 per cent of illegitimate births, some of the child murder being by the father. A paper by R.W. Malcolmson, 'Infanticide in the eighteenth century', in J.S. Cockburn (ed.), *Crime in England 1555–1800* (London, 1977), pp. 187–209, suggests a higher level in the eighteenth century, and shows that in Staffordshire infanticide and concealment cases (which the author clearly thinks were bound to be cases of child killing) formed a quarter of the homicide trials. The author points out that most of the accused's claims of stillbirths cannot be true, for the stillbirth rate would then be impossibly high.
16 An example is the correspondence in the *Scots Magazine* of 1757.
17 It was usually the minister who reported to the session the existence of a foundling, which suggests that he was the first to know of it. A minister would be the best informed in the parish on who had recently lost a child and would be able to nurse another: for this reason leaving the child at his door gave it the best prospect of survival.
18 The session's words (May 1700) were 'Which Child being now come to the length of five years and upwards, The Session thinks she may travel and shift for her Self at the begging and ordains no more to be given her.'
19 At Udny this cost the parish five shillings, a small charge compared to the support of a foundling.
20 As Chapter 2 made clear, this was unusually late in time for a session to be expressing such sentiments, which are far more typical of the seventeenth and early eighteenth century than of the 1740s.
21 For examples see Dalkeith, June 1776 and Torphichen, August 1778 and June 1779.
22 See January and February 1724, September 1725, and March 1740.
23 James Kirk (ed.), *Records of the synod of Lothian and Tweeddale* (Stair Society, Edinburgh, 1977), p. 291.
24 John Henderson, *Caithness Family History* (Edinburgh, 1884).
25 Dumfries and Galloway was another area of small lairds, and, again, some of these were responsible for a disproportionate number of pregnancies. James Murray of Conheath himself was named as father by two other women in Dumfries.

26 About 20 years after our period ends, the Reverend J.L. Buchanan commented that a woman 'if she is pregnant by a gentleman, is by no means looked down upon, but is provided in a husband with greater eclat than without forming such a connection.' J.L. Buchanan, *Travels in the Western Hebrides from 1782 to 1790* (London, 1793), p. 110. Whether such an observation was applicable in our period, or in other regions, we have no way of knowing.
27 SRO, SC 63/10/1.
28 Rosalind Mitchison, 'East Lothian as innovator in the Old Poor Law', *Transactions of the East Lothian Antiquarian and Field Naturalists Society*, vol. 19 (1987), pp. 24–7.

Conclusion

The initial, simple intent of our research was to see whether the later nineteenth-century pattern of illegitimacy in Scotland, high nationally, and particularly high in the south-west and the north-east, existed in the early modern period. This has been answered in a somewhat puzzling way. At national level illegitimacy was actually falling at the beginning of our period and remained low throughout. The regional picture is unexpected. In the south-west there was a rise from the 1750s which could well have led into the levels of the mid- and late nineteenth century; in the north-east there was no such rise. Whatever brought about the nineteenth century patterns of illegitimacy must have happened at different times in the various regions, and may well have reflected different factors.

For this book our figures were drawn entirely from rural areas and fairly small towns, and not at all from the main cities. Before 1755 the great bulk of the population was rurally based, and even by 1780 towns did not possess more than 20 per cent of the population, so the emphasis of our material is reasonably representative for Scotland as a whole. (As can be seen in *Sin in the City,* the results of later research, the picture is somewhat different in the cities of Edinburgh, Glasgow, Dundee and Aberdeen.)

T.C. Smout found for the nineteenth century that there was no ambiguity about whether couples were married or 'living in sin',[1] and we have shown that this was also true of our period, because the Kirk was determined to allow no such ambiguity. If there was not good documentary evidence of marriage a kirk session would call upon the couple to declare that they married each other. Marriage 'by habit and repute' was merely a form of evidence recognised by State courts, and, except in troubled times (e.g. during the Forty-Five), or the odd exception of Kelso, was rarely invoked. Any cohabiting couple would be reported to the kirk session, and kirk sessions establish their circumstances and status long before any reputation for being a 'married couple' could be acquired. The Church did not tolerate any so-called 'common law marriage' or 'consensual union', and only in exceptional circumstances could a couple continue in a stable but unmarried union. So the status of a birth as legitimate or illegitimate was equally plain and unambiguous.[2] Moreover, the definitions did not change, so in spite of the gap of 75 years between our material and that produced by civil registration, the figures are comparable.

The women of Scotland in our period had no reliable means of contraception or abortion; their fertility was limited but constant, and probably similar to the nineteenth century. Yet bridal pregnancy was always at a very low level, and concealment or abandonment of infants was rare. We therefore believe that illegitimacy was low primarily because the system of social control was strong, and men and women seldom had sex before marriage.

It is beyond the scope of this book to explain why illegitimacy rose in the period between the breakdown of church discipline and the start of civil registration, though some contributory trends are evident. Economic growth was exceptionally rapid in Scotland in the late eighteenth and early nineteenth century, with the textile industry creating a full-time industrial work-force. The nature of rural labour also changed, as the class of subtenants or cottars was transformed into waged labourers and farm servants.[3] There does seem to have been a general demand among men for greater freedom and independence, especially in the later eighteenth century. It informed the radical movement of the 1790s and was expressed in the emigration of the 1770s to America.[4] Edinburgh Commissary Court experienced a sharp rise in divorce cases from the 1770s onward.[5] These trends indicate changes which might lead to new patterns of sexual activity and high illegitimacy in some regions by the nineteenth century.

If pre-marital pregnancy and illegitimacy were uncommon, one might expect that women who broke the rules, or their offspring, would be all the more cruelly stigmatised. In fact, apart from that section of society where there was land to inherit, this does not appear to be so. Fordyce session in 1714 ruled that mothers as well as fathers should be named in the baptismal register 'for distinguishing Lawfull children from bastards', but since women kept their unmarried name in Scotland the child's status would still not be obvious. Even in the nineteenth century it was the complaint of those who commented on rural illegitimacy in the north-east that there was no stigma attaching to the child or to the mother.[6] A typical comment from Banffshire was that 'men seem to marry a woman who has illegitimate children without any feeling of repugnance.'[7]

The low level of bridal pregnancy means that we debunk the idea of 'fertility testing'.[8] We likewise rule out the idea of women manipulating or trapping men into marriage by sex and pregnancy, particularly as there was no tradition of 'shotgun weddings' or similar contrivances. On personal (if not economic or political matters) we have considerable evidence all through our period of study, that women were equal parties to important decisions and not subservient to men. Their attitudes, and sometimes their actual words, are on the record. Women considering marriage clearly acted, as the Kirk expected them to act, as mature and independent individuals. The legal dominance over them by fathers or husbands might force them to submit to physical violence but did not prevent them from speaking their minds. And this was true not just of wealthy women or those with a professional skill (wives of landowners and midwives for example), but at all levels of society.

Nevertheless, there was a dual standard of sexual morality, and during the nineteenth century this became more rigid. Men had the economic and political power, and for them a degree of sexual promiscuity was to be regarded as normal and acceptable. Women were labelled 'finer' and 'purer' than men, but in need of protection since their morality was constructed on the weak base of ignorance and unaroused sexuality. Any sexual experience except within marriage was, for them, a major fall from grace. On this logic was based the striving of respectable Victorians to reduce illegitimacy: societies, sermons, romantic literature and bullying by the poor law, were all aimed at persuading girls to retain their chastity, while little similar effort was aimed at the men.[9]

Yet for the eighteenth century, and even before 1700, we found a strikingly high level of 'admissions', that is of speedy acknowledgement of paternity by the men named by pregnant girls, as shown in Chapter 7. This is both a tribute to the pressure

Girls in Trouble

of the Church towards equality of treatment for the two sexes and an indicator of the value system of the period. Almost two-thirds of the men named admitted responsibility (thereby committing themselves to financial support) within a short time. Some, not yet named, even accompanied their partners to the session's enquiry. More acknowledged their paternity later. In Aberdeenshire and the north-east the admission rate ran at three-quarters of the whole. When allowance is made for men who could not be traced, men who had died and those in the army, the level of acceptance of responsibility is impressively high. There were unscrupulous and feckless men around, but most fathers of illegitimate children accepted the discipline of the Church, and the financial consequences of their behaviour. Of course, the girls still had to struggle with the practicalities of being a single parent.

It was possible to ignore or rebel against Church discipline, but the striking thing is that, except in the south-west and Ayrshire, few did so. The morality of the Church, and its methods of enforcing it, were accepted, 'internalised' by both sexes. A small minority had sex with the partner they would later marry. A larger minority, but still not a large number in the eighteenth century, fell victim to the temptations resulting from close working association and lack of supervision. Most of the latter suffered economically for this lapse, the men paying often more than half their annual wages for child support for several years, and in the women by financial problems, limited ability to work, and the burden of child care, presumably mitigated by family support. Public penance and fine hit both parents.

This conformity is more striking in that it continued through the period when couples increasingly ignored the rules of the Church on the regular conduct of marriage. The surge of irregular marriage from the 1720s, in those areas which had access to this facility (as shown in Chapter 4), shows that obedience to the orders of the Church was not automatic, and that couples distinguished between rules of basic morality and those of petty regulation.

There is little evidence in our material of a trend towards secularisation in Scotland. It is true that at the end of the eighteenth century the Church was withdrawing from the system of public penance, but that change seems to reflect a more individualist strain of theology. The struggle between evangelical religion and the more conventional adherence to a legally defined set of rights was to dominate Scottish politics in the 1830s and 1840s and force the Disruption of 1843. Even after that devastating reduction of its numbers and support, the Church of Scotland still had a dominant part to play in welfare and in the discussions on the social problems of urbanisation.[10]

However, the dogma of Calvinism had eroded, and the monolithic organisation of the Kirk had been fractured. The Church of Scotland, the Free Church and the various minor sects which had joined together to make up the United Presbyterian Church shared between them the bulk of the protestant population, but there were also Methodists, Baptists of both the Scottish and the English persuasion, Haldaneites, Congregationalists and Quakers, as well as the rare communions of Unitarians, Glassites and Irvingites. Irish immigration had drastically increased the significance of the Roman Catholic community, and, in particular, enhanced its numbers in the Lowlands, as well as having increased the episcopal component of protestantism. Fragmentation made it possible for churchmen to put the blame for what they saw as a social evil on the adherents of other bodies (though in reality many of the other sects were even stricter than the established Church.) If the inevitability of church discipline had been an element in limiting extra-marital sexual activity in the early modern period, this had ceased to be the case by the mid-nineteenth century.

But it would be unreasonably particularist to emphasise the change in the structure of the churches when society as a whole had undergone a major transformation. It had moved from a system of direct social control by lordship to one of control by economic forces and of influence, sometimes control, by organs of the State. By the 1850s as many people lived in towns as in the countryside. Most were employed in work which was based on concentrations of capital and power supply, in the form of large scale industry or of large farms. The labour needs were specific and the rewards of labour restricted, separating deeply the people who controlled work from those who supplied the labour. Certainly the Scottish economy had been expanding rapidly in the last 30 years of our study, but this was mainly an expansion within the existing structure of economic units: the farms, mills, and cottage industries. The industrial revolution, when it came, supplanted this with new units and new types of work. One's place of work and place of residence were separated, and so were the rules of social conduct applicable to each.

We are not in a position to make more than general suggestions about the very marked rise in illegitimacy in the north-east and the south-west by the later 1850s. In the north-east it was as if the clock had been turned back to the mid-seventeenth century, when over 40 per cent of first births were conceived out of wedlock and the illegitimacy ratio stood at 9.8 per cent. In Rothiemay, possessed of an exceptionally good OPR, illegitimacy began to rise after 1811, with the onset of agricultural improvement, but bridal pregnancy had started to increase in the 1770s.[11] Mothers would leave illegitimate infants, once weaned, with parents or with a sister. Children reared in the families of different parentage would see such a household structure as normal. Those able to confine their procreative life within marriage would be regarded as fortunate rather than as virtuous.[12]

In the south-west, however, illegitimacy rose before the period of agricultural improvement. The most profitable type of farming there was dairy farming, which did not need large units. Dairymaids were skilled and valued workers. The two classes of farmer and labourer were more closely related than elsewhere in Scotland.[13] What this confirms is that it was not agricultural 'improvement' as such that changed behaviour, but the nexus of human relationships and obligations.[14]

Yet the men of that region did not readily acquiesce in church discipline: the low level of 'admissions' in this area all through our period is one of its striking features. This is also the region producing most of the instances in which a woman refused to name the father of her illegitimate child. In the eighteenth century, when Galloway was the only area of lowland Scotland with any organised form of resistance to agricultural innovation and reorganisation (specifically to enclosure),[15] it stands out for the unwillingness of the population to abide by the rulings of the Church. It seems fair, therefore, to see the south-west of Scotland as an area with a long tradition of resistance to authority, and to accept that a relatively high level of illegitimacy and an unwillingness of both sexes to bring home responsibility for bastards to their fathers, was part of that resistance.

Apart from the behaviour of the south-west, Scotland's experience is important in discussing the motivation of early modern society in sexual matters. It was learning to contain sexual impulse within the narrow range of opportunity given by society,

Girls in Trouble

out of acceptance of the Church's rules. This lasted through a period of rapid economic change in the eighteenth century, but did not survive the industrial revolution.

Notes

1 T.C. Smout, 'Illegitimacy – a reply', *Scottish Journal of Sociology 2* (1977), p. 98.
2 Evidence that there was no consensual union in two parishes in the south-west during the nineteenth century appears in R.J.M. Paddock, 'Aspects of Illegitimacy in Victorian Dumfriesshire' (Unpublished Ph.D. thesis, Edinburgh, 1989).
3 The period of an upward movement in illegitimacy in the Lothians, existing for too short a period to be clear as a trend, may be the start of a longer movement and reflect these changes, but without a longer run of good figures we cannot be sure. See Alastair Orr, 'Farm labour in the Forth Valley and southern Lowlands', in T.M. Devine (ed.), *Farm Servants and Labour in Lowland Scotland, 1770–1914* (Edinburgh, 1984), p. 32, and Malcolm Gray, 'Scottish Emigration: the social impact of agrarian change in the rural Lowlands, 1775–1875', *Perspectives in American History, 7* (1973), pp. 95–174.
4 Tenants, often men of substance, were removing themselves and their families from an agricultural system where landowners had the right to their labour services. Bernard Bailyn, *Voyagers to the West* (London, 1986), pp. 517–19.
5 Leah Leneman, '"Disregarding the Matrimonial Vows" – Divorce in Eighteenth and Early Nineteenth-Century Scotland', *Journal of Social History, Vol. 30, No. 2* (Winter 1996), pp. 465–82.
6 E.g. George Seton, *The Causes of Illegitimacy* (Edinburgh, 1860); see also T.C. Smout, 'Sexual behaviour in nineteenth-century Scotland', in Peter Laslett, Karla Oosterveen and Richard M. Smith (eds.), *Bastardy and its Comparative History* (London, 1980), pp. 206–8.
7 W. Cramond, *Illegitimacy in Banffshire* (Banff, 1888), p. 49.
8 This has even acquired academic credence. Ivy Pinchbeck, 'Social Attitudes to the Problem of Illegitimacy', *British Journal of Sociology 5* (1954), pp. 309–23, claims that fertility testing was common in Scotland, but she provides no evidence for the statement.
9 J.E.D. Blaikie, *Illegitimacy, Sex and Society: North-East Scotland, 1750–1900* (Oxford, 1993), shows many of the efforts, including the Onward and Upward Society. See also Alfred C.C. List, *The two phases of the social evil* (Edinburgh, 1861). This lopsided view of sexual activity was still prevalent in the late twentieth century, as shown by a statement of the Moral Welfare Committee of the Church of Scotland in 1972, that 'the promiscuous girl' was 'the real problem'. Callum Brown, *The Social History of Religion in Scotland since 1730* (London, 1987), p. 230.
10 Brown, *Social History of Religion*, pp. 196–8.
11 Blaikie, *Illegitimacy, Sex and Society*. There is also evidence of relatively high illegitimacy in other communions in the north-east. The Catholic population of Tomintoul had an illegitimacy ratio of 16 per cent in the years 1808–11, and of 23.5 for 1817–21. By the 1840s the level was 35 per cent. Alasdair Roberts, 'Illegitimacy in Catholic Upper Banffshire', *Scottish Journal of Sociology 3* (1978–9), pp. 213–24.
12 Blaikie, *Illegitimacy, Sex and Society,* Ch. 3 gives instances of such households; Smout, in Peter Laslett, Karla Oosterveen and Richard M. Smith (eds.), *Bastardy and its Comparative History* (London, 1980), p. 206, points out that in some parts of the south-west illegitimacy appeared to be hereditary.
13 R.H. Campbell, 'Agricultural labour in the South-West', in T.M. Devine (ed.), *Farm Servants and Labour in Lowland Scotland, 1770–1914,* pp. 55–70.
14 A study of late nineteenth-century illegitimacy in two parishes in this region places it mainly among women working as farm servants. Paddock, 'Aspects of Illegitimacy'.
15 J. Leopold, 'The Levellers' revolt in Galloway in 1724', *Scottish Labour History Journal, 14* (1980), pp. 4–29.

Appendix

A List of Parishes used for Quantitative Work

These parishes form the basis of our quantification, but the KSRs of other parishes have been used to illustrate particular points. We do not cite our material by its catalogue references in the SRO because since the time of our original research many of the registers have been moved to regional archives. However, we have given the parish name, and the month and year for the information used, which will enable those who so wish to trace the register involved through SRO. In many cases the SRO still carries a microfilm copy of the material transferred.

Lothians
Cramond, Dalkeith, Pencaitland, Spott, Torphichen.

Fife
Kingsbarns, Dysart, Wemyss, Kinglassie.

Central Lowlands
Dunbarney, Dunblane, St Ninians, Falkirk, Muiravonside, Trinity Gask, Longforgan, Auchterarder, Logie, Gargunnock, Fossoway, Muthill, Forgandenny, Fintry.

Central and Eastern Highlands
Petty, Croy, Kilmadock, Alvie, Moulin, Kenmore, Blair Atholl.

Western Highlands
Kingarth, Kilmartin, Rothesay, Kilmory, Gleneray, Inveraray, Golspie, Kilfinan, Kilbrandon, Lochgoilhead, Durness.

Aberdeenshire
Longside, Belhelvie, Kemnay, Ellon, Foveran.

North-east
Grange, Fordyce, Forglen, Alves, Drainie, Banff.

Caithness
Thurso, Wattin, Olrig, Canisbay.

Ayrshire
Ayr, Kilmarnock, Kilwinning, Mauchline, Dailly, Sorn, Kirkoswald, Straiton, Dundonald, Dalrymple, Kilbirnie.

South-west
Dumfries, Westerkirk, Applegarth, Kells, Penninghame, Minnigaff, Glencairn, Wigtown, Eskdalemuir, Stranraer, Colvend, Troqueer, New Abbey.

Index

Aberdeen, 57, 111
Aberdeenshire, 4, 32, 75, 77–8, 83, 85, 127
   admissions in, 107
   in the nineteenth century, 75
Aberdour, 109
abortion, 2, 81, 122
   attempts, 106, 109, 110
Aboyne, Earl of, 117
admissions of paternity, 83, 102, 107, 123, 124, 125
adultery, 10, 66, 99
   'notour', 43
affinity, 42–3; *see also* incest
agricultural revolution, 2, 28, 74
agriculture, change in, 28–9, 97
Aikenhead, Thomas, 30
aliment, of bastards, 79–80, 107
Alves, 79, 114, 127
Alvie, 78, 127
America, 29, 123
Angus, 3
Annals of the Parish, 35
Anstruther, 34, 39, 45
anti-clericalism, 30–1
appearances, public, 16, 17, 81
Applegarth, 127
Argyll, Synod of, 9
aristocracy, 6–7, 13, 23, 25
Arnot, Hugh, 34
assessment, 27
Auchterarder, 127
Auld, William, 35
Ayr, 57, 59, 66, 99, 127
Ayrshire, 3, 26, 36, 57, 75–8, 84–5, 87, 88, 127
   admissions in, 107, 124
   in the nineteenth century, 75

Banff, 62, 66, 101, 108, 116, 127
Banffshire, 4, 26
   illegitimacy in, 2, 82, 89, 123
Bannerman, Patrick, 31
banns, *see* proclamation
baptism, 24, 71, 74, 84, 106, 117, 119

Barclay, John, 58–9
baron courts, 13
bed-sharing, 92, 94, 95, 97, 104
Belhelvie, 49, 94, 101, 108, 109, 127
bestiality, 98–9
bigamy, 55, 64–5, 67
birth rates, 73
   English, 74
   Scottish, 74
bishops, 7, 11
blacks, 100, 117
Blaikie, George, 60
Blair Atholl, 42, 97–8, 100, 114, 127
bonnet lairds, 25–6
Borders, 3, 15, 26, 55, 71
Boswell, James, 94
breach of contract, 45–6
Brodie, Alexander, 6
burghs, 24
Burns, Robert, 34, 35
Burt, Edmund, 104, 105
Bute, 26

Caithness, 4, 75–8, 79, 84–5, 89, 127
   gentry in, 26, 117
   in the nineteenth century, 75
   physical penalties in, 24
Caithness, 9th Earl of, 47
Calder, 48
Calvinism, 5, 30, 124
Cambuslang, 32–3, 38
Cameron, 24
Canisbay, 47, 50, 86, 100–1, 109, 114, 117, 127
Canongate, irregular marriage in, 58
Carlyle, Alexander, 34
Catechism, Shorter, 35
Catholicism, Roman, 9
Central Lowlands, 3, 26, 57, 68, 75–6, 78, 85, 107, 127
   in the nineteenth century, 75
chapmen, 16
Charles I, 10, 24
child molestation, 99
Church,

Index

Episcopal, 4, 7, 57
Episcopalian, 11, 12
Free, 124
 of England, 13, 14, 57
 of Scotland, 1, 2, 7, 10–11, 13, 15, 20, 22–3, 24, 27, 30, 31, 35–6, 115, 119, 124
Presbyterian, 11, 17
Roman Catholic, 4, 24, 39, 68, 124
see also dissent; presbyterian system
church courts, 7, 83
church discipline, 3
 disintegration of, 124
civic humanism, 29–30
Civil War, *see* Great Rebellion
clan chiefs, 22
Clanny, Hugh, 59
Cockburn, John, of Ormiston, 29
Coldstream, irregular marriage in, 63
Colvend, 127
Commissary Court, 23, 43, 123
Commissioners of Supply, 7, 12, 13
Commonwealth period, 14
communion, 5
Confession of Faith, 5, 6
 (1560), 6
 (1690), 42
Confession, Westminster, 32, 33
conformity, 124
Connacher case (1755), 55
consensual unions, 79, 122
consent, parental, 41
consignation money, 40, 48, 84
contraception, 81, 120, 122
contumacy, 115–16
cottars, 21, 123
Counter Reformation, 23
courtship, 82, 91, 93
Covenant (1638), 6
covenant theology, 5–6
Cramond, 11, 58, 59, 61, 68, 87, 92, 112, 113, 117, 119, 127
Cramond, W., 123, 126
Creech, William, 32
crime, concepts of, 23
Croy, 100, 127
Cumbernauld, irregular marriage in, 59

Dailly, 50, 78, 98, 101, 127
Dalkeith, 36, 54, 58, 62, 68, 87, 92, 112, 113, 117, 119, 127
Dalrymple, 36, 127
Daviot (Inverness-shire), 113

denial,
 of paternity, 46, 107–9
 of pregnancy, 106–7, 111–12
desertion, 43, 50
Disruption, of the Church (1843), 124
dissent, 36, 134; *see also* Original Secession; Relief Church
divorce, 43–4, 52, 66, 99, 123, 126
domestic industry, 28–9, 81; *see also* linen industry
Domestic Medicine, 90
'domestic revolution', 24
Douglas, Patrick, 60
Drainie, 45, 107, 111, 127
Drake, Thomas, 59
dual standard, 123
Dumbarton, 24
Dumfries, 4, 53, 57, 59, 61, 69, 71, 109, 117, 127
 Synod of, 146
Dumfriesshire, 78, 120, 124
Dunbar,
 presbytery of, 41
 battle of, 17
Dunbarney, 69, 127
Dunblane, 127
Dundee, 46, 57, 61, 68, 69, 71
Dundonald, 98, 127
Dunkeld, 99
Durness, 127
Dysart, 48, 58, 59, 62, 66, 69, 95–6, 99, 102, 109, 110, 111–12, 113, 115, 127

East Linton, 69
East Lothian, 26, 89
economic growth, 122, 125
Eddleston, 112
Edinburgh, 33, 41
 flight to, 109
 General Session of, 9
 irregular marriage in, 57
 Royal Society of, 33
eldership, 7, 10, 101–2
Elgin, 36
Elliots of Minto, 25
Ellon, 36, 112, 114, 127
emigration, 123
England, 3, 12, 15, 35, 39, 94
 flight to, 44
 illegitimacy in, 2, 14, 79, 81, 102, 120
 irregular marriage in, 57
 see also Union (1707)
Enlightenment, 26, 29–30, 33, 35

129

Girls in Trouble

Eskdalemuir, 44, 61, 127
Essex, 81, 120
Evangelical party, 124; *see also* Popular party
excommunication, 7, 43, 67, 115

Falkirk, 127
farm service, 124, 126
fertility, legitimate, 81
fertility testing, 82, 123
festivals, 96
Fife, 3, 26, 57, 68, 75–6, 78, 84–5, 88, 107, 127
    in the nineteenth century, 75
Fintry, 127
First Book of Discipline, 41
Fletcher, Andrew of Saltoun, 16
Flinn, M.W., 74, 89
Forbes, Benjamin, 118
Fordyce, 111, 123, 127
Forfar, 54
Forgandenny, 60, 84, 114–15, 127
Forglen, 78, 113, 127
fornication, 2, 23
    antenuptial, 47
    exposure of, 72
Fossoway, 48, 74, 113, 127
foundlings, 112–13, 120
Foveran, 36, 48, 99, 106, 109, 118, 127
France, 39
    illegitimacy in, 42
franchises, 12

Gaelic, 4, 8, 9
Galloway, 4, 16, 26, 41, 78, 82, 109, 120, 124
Gargunnock, 127
General Assembly, 7, 12, 31, 33, 83–5
    Act of, 34
    Commission of, 9, 83
gentry, 25, 102, 116–19, 121
    women, 81, 102, 108, 123
gestation time, opinions on, 83, 90
Glasgow, 33, 70
    irregular marriage in, 57, 62
Glencairn, 127
Glenelg, Synod of, 9, 98
Gleneray, 127
Golspie, 99, 127
Grange, 36, 50, 87–8, 109, 112, 127
Great Rebellion, 12, 13
Greenock, irregular marriage in, 57
Gretna, irregular marriage in, 1, 58

Grierson, John, 60

Hair, P.E.H., 90
Hajnal system of marriage, 42, 51
Hamilton, Gavin, 35
Highland Society, 33
Highlands, 8, 9, 12, 15, 16, 21–2, 27, 82, 108
    agriculture in, 22
    Central and Eastern region, 4, 75–6, 85, 87, 107, 112, 127
    disorder in, 16
    food shortage in, 27
    Western region, 4, 57, 75–7, 85, 96, 107, 108, 112, 127
hiring fairs, 13
Home family, 42
homosexuality, 98
Hoskins, W.G., 24
housing, 24–5
humanitarianism, 34–5
Hume, Baron David, 111
Hume, David, 31, 34

illegitimacy, 70, 88, 91, 105, 120, 122, 123
    regional variations in, 76–7
illegitimacy rate, 73
illegitimacy ratio, 37, 73–4, 81
    English, 14, 75, 81, 88
    in the nineteenth century, 80, 124
'improvement', 28–9, 46–7
    agricultural, 28–9
    see also agricultural revolution
incapacity,
    mental, 101
    physical, 100
incest, 42, 51–2, 67, 97
individualism, 22–3, 29
industrial revolution, 26, 124
industrialisation, 123
industries, 20; *see also* linen industry
inequality, sexual, 24, 51, 123
infant mortality, 81
infanticide, 24, 34, 110–12, 120
    in England, 112, 120
    see also pregnancy, concealment of
Ingram, M., 18, 104, 105
Inveraray, 62, 127
Inveresk, 110
Ireland, 53–4
    flight to, 109
    migration from, 124

Index

Jacobitism, 11, 55; *see also* rising
James VI, 25, 41
Jamieson, William, 60
Jockey and Maggie's Courtship, 34
Johnston, Charles, 60
jus primae noctis, 94
Justices of the Peace, 7, 13, 25, 30, 67, 80
Justiciary, Court of, 12, 99

Kells, 96
Kelso, 59, 60–1, 63, 66, 67, 69–70, 122
Kemnay, 78, 127
Kenmore, 42, 51, 80, 86–7, 91, 113, 116, 127
Kennoway, 113
Kilbirnie, 78, 88, 127
Kilbrandon, 45, 53, 127
Kilfinan, 93, 95, 96, 97, 127
Kilmadock, 127
Kilmarnock, 45–6, 84, 88, 106, 127
Kilmartin, 20, 65, 70, 78, 96, 127
Kilmory, 47–8, 49, 127
Kilwinning, 98, 127
Kingarth, 102, 127
Kinglassie, 46, 61, 85–6, 107, 114, 127
Kingsbarns, 61, 87, 111, 127
Kirk session registers, 15, 111
Kirk sessions, 1, 7, 44, 70, 72–3, 78, 82–3, 91, 107, 118, 122
    attitudes of, 113
Kirkcudbright, Stewartry of, 89
Kirkoswald, 107, 127
Knight, Christopher, 58
Knockando, 89
Knox, John, 5
Kussmaul, Ann, 105

labourers, 21, 24
lairds, 26; *see also* bonnet lairds; gentry; landowners
Lamberton toll, irregular marriage at, 58
Lanarkshire, 3, 26
Lancashire, 81
landowners, 15, 20, 22, 25–7, 116, 119
    hostility to clergy, 31–2
landowning, 20, 45, 49
Laslett, Peter, 18, 79, 82, 89–90, 126
Levine, David, 79, 89–90
Leviticus XVIII, 42, 43
linen industry, 28, 81–2, 123
Linlithgow, 113
literacy, 65, 112
local government, 12

Lochgoilhead, 62, 100, 127
Logie, 74, 86, 127
Longforgan, 92, 127
Longside, 54, 84, 99, 127
Lothian and Tweeddale, Synod of, 41, 116
Lothians, 3, 21, 57, 68, 75–6, 81, 85, 107, 112, 127
    in the nineteenth century, 123
Lowlands, 8, 12, 20–2
    agriculture in, 21, 91
    law and order in, 25

MacKintosh, William of Borlum, 28–9
Malcolmson, R.W., 102
Man, Isle of, 3, 13
marital disharmony, 50–1
Marnock, 89
marriage, 1, 40
    by habit and repute, 53, 62–3, 122
    civil law of, 40, 44, 70
    contract of, 46
    handfast, 54, 71
    in England, civil, 57
    in south Germany, 82
    in Sweden, 82
    irregular, 1, 53–71, 82, 124
    legislation on, 42, 53, 55, 57
    penalties for irregular marriage, 71
    promise of, 44–6, 49–50, 53, 93
    regular, 40, 53
    verba de futuro, 53
    verba de praesenti, 53, 54
Marriage Act (English), Hardwicke's (1753), 57, 70
Marriage Bill (Scottish) (1755), 57
Marrow of Modern Divinity, The, 32
Martin, Martin, 19, 71
maternity testing, 107, 111
Mauchline, 67, 109, 127
Mearns, 3
midwives, 86–7, 94, 107, 111, 113, 123
migration, 29, 35
miners, 13
ministers, 26, 101
    episcopalian, 16, 58–9
Minnigaff, 127
mobility, 29; *see also* migration
Moderate party, 30, 33–4
Monro, Alexander, 30
Montauban, 39
Montrose, 109
Moray, 4
Moulin, 65, 127

131

Girls in Trouble

Mowat, Samuel, 58
Muiravonside, 58, 66, 67, 74, 127
Murray, Thomas, 60
Murrays of Scone, 25
Mushet, Gilbert, 59
Muthill, 59, 60, 61, 68, 74, 127

Nairnshire, 4
Netherlands, flight to, 15
New Abbey, 68, 108, 111, 127
New Monkland, 42
north-east region, 4, 32, 68, 71, 75, 77, 78–9, 83, 85, 88, 122, 127
   admissions in, 107
   in the nineteenth century, 75, 122
Northern Isles, 3

oath, 23, 86, 90, 103, 108, 119
Ogle, Thomas, 59
Olrig, 127
OPR (Old Parish Register), *see* parish registers
Original Secession, 12, 32
OSA, see *Statistical Account of Scotland*
Oswald, James, 31

parishes, 44
parish registers, 8, 14, 84, 88
   English, 14
parish schools, 7
Parliament,
   of Great Britain, 32
   of Scotland, 20, 28, 40
paternity, 123–4; *see also* denial
Paterson, David, 60
patronage, 32
peasant society, 21–2
penance, public, 16, 72, 104, 124; *see also* appearances
Pencaitland, 44, 48, 68, 98, 111, 127
Penninghame, 99, 127
Penpont, 86
Perth, 69
Perthshire, 3
Petty, 87, 103, 127
Pittenweem, 30
polygamy, 65–7
Poor Law, English, 14
poor relief, 8, 27–8, 31, 102
   funds for, 27, 31
Popular party, 33
population growth, 22
predestination, 5, 30

pregnancy, 72, 89, 91, 103
   concealment of, 34, 68, 100–1
   duration of, 108
   pre-marital, 37, 67, 68, 73, 82, 84–7, 103, 122, 123, 124
   pre-marital in England, 90
presbyterian system, 7–10, 17
presbyteries, 7–9, 31, 43, 61, 62, 66, 68, 75, 106, 110, 111
Privy Council, Scottish, 28, 40
proclamation of banns, 40, 45–6, 48, 71, 85
prostitution, 116

Quaife, G.R., 18, 104
Quakers, 124

rape, 1, 41, 98, 99, 100, 104
Ratho, 117
Reformation, 5, 7, 23
regions, 3; *see also* Aberdeenshire; Ayrshire; Caithness; Central Lowlands; Fife; Highlands, Central and Eastern; Highlands, Western; Lothians; North-east; South-west
registration, civil, 2, 122
relapse, 117; *see also* repeating
Relief Church, 12, 32, 33
repeating, 78–9
resiling from marriage, 47–8
resistance, to authority, 83, 155
Restoration period, 12, 23, 25
Revolution (1689), 11, 32, 83
rising,
   of 1715, 12, 23, 32
   of 1745, 23
Roman Catholics, 17, 68
Ross and Cromarty, 2, 89
Rothesay, 59, 70, 102, 117, 127
Rothiemay, 89, 124

St Ninians, 59, 64, 101, 113, 116, 127
'scandalous carriage', 2, 72, 91–2
Scots law, 23; *see also* marriage
secularisation, 124
Selkirk, 119
sermons, 31
servants, 81, 94, 117
Session, Court of, 13, 43
sheriff court, 28
sheriffs, 13
Sinclair, Sir John, 26, 32, 74
Smith, Adam, 30
Smith, Richard M., 18, 89–90, 126

132

Index

Smout, T.C., 6, 51, 71, 89, 91, 104, 122, 124
soldiers, 15–16, 61, 66
Somerset, 13, 94, 96
Sorn, 48, 49, 50, 127
South Leith, 57, 67
south-west, 57, 68, 75, 78, 82, 85, 88, 122, 124, 127
   admissions in, 107, 124
   in the nineteenth century, 75, 78, 122
Spott, 36, 62, 106, 127
Statistical Account of Scotland (OSA), 34, 74, 89
Stewart, David, of Garth, 103–4
Stewart, John, 60
stigma,
   of bastardy, 123
   of unmarried motherhood, 103–4, 123
Stirlingshire, 3
   synod of, 31
Stone, Lawrence, 18
Straiton, 36, 127
Strange, David, 59–60, 68, 69
Stranraer, 44, 63, 127
Sunday observance, 11, 35, 37, 50, 106, 115
support of bastards, 79–80, 124; *see also* aliment
synods, 9, 66, 83

Terling, 89
'testificats', 15, 29, 53, 102
   forgery of, 59, 61, 67
Thurso, 47, 84, 92–3, 102, 108, 116–17, 127
Timperley, L., 26
Toleration Act (1712), 12, 31, 55
Tomintoul, 126
Torphichen, 44, 59, 87, 109, 111, 112, 114, 127
Torthorwald, 89
towns, 29, 36; *see also* Edinburgh
   urbanisation, 122
Tranent, 14
transport system, 29
trilapse, 116
Trinity Gask, 80, 127

Troqueer, 44–5, 53, 58, 61, 63, 64–5, 69, 70, 127
Turriff, 113

Ulster, 15
unemployment, 97
Union (1707), 11, 13, 22–3, 25, 31, 32
Unitarians, 46
urbanisation, 39, 124; *see also* migration

vagrants, 16

Wallace, Robert, 33
Wamphray, 78
Wattin, 102, 106, 108, 116, 127
Webster, Alexander, census by (1755), 73–4, 78, 89
weddings, 13
Wemyss, 58, 65, 80, 84–5, 86, 93, 95–6, 98, 101, 109, 110, 117–18, 127
Wemyss, Earls of, 117–18
Westerkirk, 78–9, 119, 127
Western Isles, 3
Westminster Directory, 40
wet-nursing, 28
Whitefield, George, 32
wife-beating, 50–1
Wigtown, 49, 109, 127
Wigtownshire, 89
William III, 11
Williamson, David, 60
Wiltshire, 13
witchcraft, 23, 30
Witherspoon, John, 30, 33–4
Wodrow, Robert, 41
women, 123
   as witness, 23–4
   criminalisation of, 23
   independence of, 123
   occupations of, 24, 96
Wrightson, Keith, 14, 81, 89
Wrigley, E.A., 88, 89, 90

Yester, 17, 112